TABLE OF CONTENTS

Top 20 Test Taking Tips

1. Carefully follow all the test registration procedures
2. Know the test directions, duration, topics, question types, how many questions
3. Setup a flexible study schedule at least 3-4 weeks before test day
4. Study during the time of day you are most alert, relaxed, and stress free
5. Maximize your learning style; visual learner use visual study aids, auditory learner use auditory study aids
6. Focus on your weakest knowledge base
7. Find a study partner to review with and help clarify questions
8. Practice, practice, practice
9. Get a good night's sleep; don't try to cram the night before the test
10. Eat a well balanced meal
11. Know the exact physical location of the testing site; drive the route to the site prior to test day
12. Bring a set of ear plugs; the testing center could be noisy
13. Wear comfortable, loose fitting, layered clothing to the testing center; prepare for it to be either cold or hot during the test
14. Bring at least 2 current forms of ID to the testing center
15. Arrive to the test early; be prepared to wait and be patient
16. Eliminate the obviously wrong answer choices, then guess the first remaining choice
17. Pace yourself; don't rush, but keep working and move on if you get stuck
18. Maintain a positive attitude even if the test is going poorly
19. Keep your first answer unless you are positive it is wrong
20. Check your work, don't make a careless mistake

Antepartal Period

Normal Pregnancies

Subjective signs and symptoms of pregnancy

Amenorrhea

Amenorrhea, absence of menstruation, is one of the first signs of pregnancy. Most women menstruate on a 28-day cycle with ovulation occurring at about day 14 of the cycle. The ovum remains fertile for 12 to 24 hours. For conception to occur, intercourse must take place within 5 to 6 days before or including the day of ovulation. Sperm remain most fertile in the female reproductive tract for 24 hours. Fertilization (conception) usually takes place in the fallopian tube, and during the first 14 days (pre-embryonic stage), cell division and cell multiplication occur, forming an inner layer (blastocyst) and outer layer (trophoblast). If fertilization of the egg does not occur, the uterine lining begins to shed and menstruation occurs on about day 23. However, if the trophoblast attaches to the endometrium of the uterus (implantation), usually 7 to 10 days after fertilization, the uterine lining thickens, and the trophoblast cells grow into the lining. The placenta forms and hormonal changes associated with pregnancy prevent menstruation.

Nausea and vomiting, and fatigue

Human chorionic gonadotropin (hCG) levels increase, and carbohydrate metabolism changes, resulting in nausea, especially in the morning. This "morning sickness" (which actually can occur at any time during the day) usually occurs 6 weeks after the last menstrual period and lasts for 6 to 12 weeks, although it may be prolonged in some women. During the first trimester, the body goes through many changes as the placenta forms and the embryo grows into the fetus, causing exhaustion that is not relieved by sleeping or rest. The mother should rest as much as possible, modifying activities. Symptoms subside by the second trimester.

Breast changes and abdominal enlargement

Breast changes (growth, engorgement, tenderness, prominent veins, stretch marks, itching) often begin to occur even before the first missed period. Hormone changes promote growth of the ductal system to prepare the breasts for milk production. Breasts usually grow about a cup size. At 6 to 8 weeks, the nipples begin to enlarge and Montgomery's tubercles (bumps around the areola) become more obvious. Discomfort usually recedes after the first trimester. A support bra may help relieve discomfort. Progressive abdominal enlargement associated with amenorrhea is characteristic of pregnancy. Little change is evident during the first trimester as the fundal height remains within the pelvis, but the abdomen enlarges as the uterus grows and fundal height moves upward.

Urinary frequency and quickening

During the first trimester, the growing uterus presses on the bladder, causing frequent urge to urinate, and increased vascularization increases volume of urinary output. Symptoms recede as the uterus rises into the abdomen during the second trimester but return when the uterus descends again into the pelvic area during the third trimester. Movement of the fetus is usually detected at 18 to 20 weeks after the LMP in a primigravida or 16 weeks in a multigravida. Quickening is often described as a "fluttering" within the abdomen.

Objective changes

Pregnancy tests

Pregnancy should be verified by a positive pregnancy test:

- Urine tests: All tests measure human chorionic gonadotropin (hCG). Laboratory tests, such as hemagglutination-inhibition test and latex agglutination test, are 95 to 98 percent accurate at about 2 weeks after the first missed period. Home urine tests may detect pregnancy within a day of a missed period, but most are more accurate at 1 to 2 weeks after a missed period. False negatives are more common than false positives.
- Serum tests: These tests are more accurate than urine tests as they detect a sub-unit of hCG, so they may detect pregnancy even before a missed period. Additionally, monitoring of progesterone levels may help to determine if a pregnancy is viable as levels >25 ng/mL suggest viability and levels <5 ng/mL are inconsistent with viability.
- Ultrasound: The gestational sac can be seen transabdominally 5 to 6 weeks after the beginning of the LMP and transvaginally at 3 to 4 weeks gestation

Fetal heart tones

Fetal heart tones are usually heard at about 20 weeks gestation with a fetoscope, although they may be heard much earlier with Doppler. The heartbeat has a distinctive galloping sound, more distinct as the fetus develops. Additionally, the Doppler may pick up the maternal heartbeat as well as the sound of arterial blood flow and placental blood flow (a whooshing sound). In some cases, artifacts (popping, crackling) may be heard, although using gel on the abdomen reduces artifacts. In early pregnancy, the fetal heart tones may be heard most easily above the symphysis pubis, but later, finding the heart tones depends on the size and position of the fetus. Heart tones are easier to hear through the fetus's back, below the shoulder, so palpating the fetus to ascertain position, placing the fetoscope firmly against the skin, and moving the fetoscope slowly can help to locate heart tones. Auscultation should be done between contractions.

Fetal heart rate—Tachycardia and bradycardia

Fetal heart rate usually varies with accelerations and decelerations. Fetal reactivity (accelerated fetal heart rate with fetal activity) begins at about 32 week's gestation. Heart rate often increases for periods of 20 to 40 minutes. Causes for accelerated or decelerated fetal heart rate include the following:

- Tachycardia: Tachycardia is defined as an accelerated heart rate >160 for ≥10 minutes. In severe tachycardia, the heart rate is >180. Transient tachycardia occurs for <10 minutes and is usually not significant. Tachycardia may result from early fetal hypoxia, prematurity, medications (such as terbutaline), fetal infection, maternal fever, and anxiety.

- Bradycardia: Bradycardia is defined as a decelerated heart rate <120 for ≥10 minutes. In severe bradycardia, the heart rate is <80. Bradycardia at 100 to 119 is usually not significant, but bradycardia may indicate heart block or placentae abruptio. Uterine contractions slow fetal heart rate because of compression of the head affecting cerebral blood flow, compression of the myometrial vessels of the uterus, and/or occlusion of the umbilical cord causing fetal hypertension or hypoxemia, Medications (such as narcotics and oxytocin) and epidural anesthesia may cause decreased heart rate as well.

Fundal height

The uterine fundus (curvature at the top) can be palpated above the symphysis pubis by about 10 to 12 weeks gestation, and fundal height can be used to estimate duration of gestation and growth of the fetus. Starting at about week 16 gestation and lasting until week 36, the fundal height (from top of symphysis pubis to top of fundus) measured in centimeters usually corresponds to the weeks of gestation, so 18 cm is consistent with 18 weeks gestation in a pregnancy with a normal single fetus. At 20 weeks (20 cm), the fundus is usually at the umbilicus. After 36 weeks, the fundal height may increase slowly or decrease as the head engages in preparation for delivery. If the baby is lying across the abdomen, the fundal height may be lower than expected, and a breech presentation usually results in increased fundal height. Multiple births result in a markedly increased fundal height.

Maternal psychosexual changes

First trimester (1-13 weeks): The first trimester can be considered a time of psychosocial crisis. The woman can experience a period of stress and anxiety, which can have a profound impact on her relationship with her partner or husband. Fears of miscarriage are not unusual. These concerns by the mother can be minimized by her partner's or husband's involvement in the pregnancy, such as by accompanying his partner or wife to Lamaze classes and prenatal visits.

Second trimester (14-26 weeks): Social myths and taboos, mostly unsubstantiated, may interfere with intimacy (particularly sexual) between the mother and her partner or husband. The mother's self-perceived body image due to an expanding abdomen and weight gain may affect her self-esteem. During this time the clinician can intervene and counsel the couple on any restrictions associated with sexual relations.

Third trimester (27-42 weeks): There is generally a decline in sexual interest in the mother during this period. The woman's perceived body habitus may make her feel awkward, unattractive, and uncomfortable, leading to intimacy problems between her and her partner or husband. The couple may avoid engaging in sexual intercourse fearing labor induction, bleeding, or pain. The couple feels vulnerable at this period, and it is critical that the clinician asks the couple about their intimacy in order to lead to discussion and reassurance.

Postpartal period: Estrogen and progesterone levels drop, causing vaginal atrophy. This combined with the vaginal and perineal trauma due to the childbirth process may make intercourse uncomfortable for the pair. Healing lacerations or episiotomy and breastfeeding, along with exhaustion caused by the attention the newly arrived baby requires, may cause further problems with the relationship

Paternal psychosexual changes

First trimester (1-13 weeks): The father may feel initial excitement or concern but then begin to feel left out as the mother gets more attention. He may not understand the mother's mood swings and may resent changes in sexual activity. Fathers often fantasize about an older child (playing ball with a child) rather than an infant who may not seem real at this point.

Second trimester (14-26 weeks): While coming to terms with the pregnancy, the father may feel more connection if he goes with his partner to the doctor, listens to the fetal heartbeat, and sees the ultrasound. The father may have anxiety about his role and the expectations of the mother. If the mother is demanding of attention, he may become resentful and seek reasons to be away from home. Sexual desire may increase or decrease. The father begins to examine his relationship with his own father and to determine what type of father he wants to be.

Third trimester (27-42 weeks): This can be a time of happiness and excitement or growing detachment, depending on father's development in the first two trimesters. The father may experience growing concern about labor, delivery, and the wellbeing of the fetus. He may feel more involved if participating in classes, shopping for the baby, and actively planning for parenthood. Some fathers develop physical symptoms (couvade), such as insomnia, depression, and backache.

Postpartal Period: In some ways, this period mirrors that of the third trimester. Those fathers who felt positive then continue to do so and those who felt detached sometimes feel even more detached. The father experiences a number of concerns regarding the financial responsibilities of rearing a child, the child's need for care, inadequate sleep, lack of intimacy, and concerns about the child's future.

Developmental tasks of becoming parents

<u>Ambivalence to acceptance</u>
Almost all mothers have feelings of ambivalence about the challenges of parenthood, and these feelings are normal and healthy, representing a transitional stage leading to acceptance. Areas of concern include the following:

- Changing body image/sexuality: Weight gain, varicose veins, growing abdomen, stretch marks, and breast changes may cause the mother to fear she is no longer attractive.
- Labile moods: Hormonal and body changes can lead to rapid mood swings and emotional outbursts that may affect relationships, especially if the partner is unprepared.
- Personality changes: Pregnancy often results in a tendency toward introversion with the mother requiring more rest and personal time, and this can lead to conflicts.

If the pregnancy was unintended, the mother may especially resent the pregnancy and consider abortion, leading to feelings of guilt. Many mothers are able to work through these issues and reach acceptance, especially by the third trimester when pregnancy is obvious, and people are often more solicitous and supportive. However, this is also a time of concern for the fetus.

Preparation of siblings

Preparation of siblings prior to the birth of an infant can decrease anxiety and sibling rivalry by helping the children feel as though they are participants in the process and are valued. Children should be prepared for physical changes in the mother, changing family dynamics, and infant care. Formal classes may be available for children (3-12) to help them identify and express their concerns and teach them about pregnancy and childcare. Booklets, books, and videos are also available. The parent/teacher may use dolls to demonstrate childcare and allow the children to practice holding and caring for the baby. When possible, children should have contact with an infant, such as that of a friend or family member. Children may help to decorate the infant's room or prepare a "welcome" gift, such as a drawing or toy. Children should be told who will care for them during labor and delivery and should visit the mother and infant as soon after delivery as possible.

Preparation of grandparents

Grandparents may vary widely in their feelings about a pregnancy. For example, the parents of a pregnant adolescent may feel anger and despair while the parents of a mature married parent may be thrilled. Grandparents can provide significant support and should be included in planning early in the pregnancy, but the parents should keep clear boundaries when it comes to decision-making. In some cases, there may be conflicts between the grandparents and the parents regarding religious or cultural practices. While it may be difficult to confront these issues, it's better to deal with them during the pregnancy than after delivery. The parents should state their desires and plans openly, giving their reasons. Grandparents may benefit from classes or a review of current standards and practices in relation to pregnancy, delivery, and breastfeeding.

Health promotion

Rest

A mother often feels fatigued and must ensure she gets adequate rest. Fatigue is especially pronounced during the first trimester, usually eases in the second, and returns in the third. Strategies to increase rest include the following:

- Increase nighttime sleep to 8 to 10 hours by going to bed earlier or sleeping later.
- Experiment with different positions during sleep, but avoid lying on the stomach because this will be uncomfortable as the uterus grows. Using pillows to support the body may relieve discomfort.
- Take rest breaks or short naps during the daytime.
- Change work/social schedule by working fewer hours if possible or eliminating unnecessary meetings, activities, or social events.
- Ask for help.
- Exercise daily, such as walking.
- Eat a healthy diet and drink ample fluids.
- Activities of daily living—Dressing and bathing
- Activities of daily living during pregnancy are explained below:
- Bathing - Because of increased perspiration and vaginal discharge, pregnant women should bathe daily and may shower or take a tub bath as desired throughout pregnancy. It may be difficult for a woman to get safely in and out of a tub during the

third trimester, so she may need assistance, tub mats, and safety bars. Tub bathing is contraindicated if the woman is experiencing vaginal bleeding or the membranes have ruptured.

- Dressing - Generally, clothing should be comfortable and non-constrictive. Women excited about pregnancy often begin wearing maternity clothes earlier than women who want to hide pregnancy or feel negatively about it. Girdles are not advised unless the woman has a large pendulous abdomen, but girdles should never be constrictive about the legs as they may decrease peripheral circulation. As pregnancy progresses, women often choose clothing that is easy to get on and off.
- Exercising - Moderate exercise, such as walking, should be done for 30 minutes daily. Supine exercises should be avoided during the 2nd and 3rd trimesters because this position decreases maternal cardiac output and uterine circulation. Aerobic exercises should be modified, and exercises that require balance (gymnastics, horseback riding, skiing) should be avoided. Generally pulse rate during exercise should not be >140.
- Grooming - Pregnant women often experience an increase in acne because of hormonal changes but should avoid cleansing preparations that contain salicylic acid or anti-aging compounds with retinoids. Women should avoid hair dye and permanent waves because some of the chemicals are teratogenic, especially during the first trimester. Henna is a natural product that is safe. Lemon juice can be used to lighten facial hair rather than bleach products. Soy products may increase melasma because of estrogenic properties. Chemical hair removers and sunscreen products are generally safe for pregnant women. Most makeup is safe except for those that contain retinol or salicylic acid.
- Traveling - If a pregnant woman is healthy with no fetal complications, travel is usually not restricted; however, long automobile trips should be avoided in favor of air or train travel. If traveling by car, the woman should get out and walk for 10 minutes at least every 2 hours. She should wear both a lap belt, positioned under the abdomen and across the upper thighs and shoulder strop positioned between the breasts. Flying is acceptable until week 36 but is contraindicated with obstetric complications, placental abnormalities, or increased risk of premature delivery.
- Working - Work/employment that requires prolonged standing or demanding physical activities is associated with increased premature delivery, so work should be evaluated on an individual basis. Women should avoid working with fetotoxic hazards/chemicals and may need reassignment. In the third trimester, balance is impaired, and this may be a consideration for some jobs. One of the biggest problems associated with working is fatigue, and the woman must try to find ways to get adequate rest, such as taking regular breaks or reducing hours.

<u>Exercises in preparation for childbirth</u>

The pregnant woman can benefit from a number of specific exercises, but they should be done slowly, usually in sets of 5, being careful to avoid strain. Exercises to improve muscle tone and reduce anxiety in preparation for childbirth are discussed below:

- Pelvic tilt - Pelvic tilt strengthens both muscles in the lower back and lower abdomen, reducing back strain. Pelvic rocking is best done in the supine position with feet flat on the floor, but it can also be done on hands and knees, standing against a wall, or sitting in a chair.

- Abdominal tightening - This exercise involves pulling the abdominal muscles tight while exhaling. This exercise is most easily practiced while lying supine with feet flat on the floor.
- Partial sit-ups - Partial sit-ups strengthen abdominal muscles. The woman should lie in supine position with knees flexed and feet flat on the floor, stretching arms toward the knees while lifting the head and neck.
- Thigh stretching - Sitting in a cross-legged position stretches the muscles in the inner thighs, facilitating the birth process.

Activities of daily living—Kegel exercises

Kegel exercises strengthen the pelvic floor muscles, which cross the floor of the pelvis and attach to the pubic bone and coccyx. The urethra, rectum and vagina all open through the pelvic floor muscles, which support the pelvic organs. Strengthening these muscles helps prevent stress incontinence and childbirth-related disorders, such as uterine prolapse, rectocele, and cystocele.

- Caution: Avoid holding the breath or tightening the abdominal or buttocks muscles during pelvic floor exercises.
- Procedure: Tighten and squeeze the muscles about the rectum, vagina, and urethra and try to "lift" them inside as though trying to stop from passing gas and urine. Hold. Relax. Rest a few seconds. Repeat.
- Schedule: Exercises should be done at least 3 times daily. They may be done while lying down in the morning and evening and while sitting midday.
    - Initially: Tighten 1 second, relax 5. Repeat 5 to 10 times.
    - Later: Tighten 5 seconds or longer and relax 10. Repeat 10 times.

Nutritional needs

Dietary reference intakes

The nutrition of the mother has a profound effect on the developing embryo/fetus. Caloric needs vary widely depending on the mother's age, size, weight, metabolism, and general health. Energy needs of the mother usually remain stable during the first trimester but an added 300 kilocalories a day are needed during the second and third trimester for a singleton and 600 kilocalories a day for twins. Recommended dietary intake for pregnant women includes the following:

- A (μg/d) - 750-770
- C (mg/d) - 80-85
- D (μg/d) - ≥5
- E (mg/d) - 15
- K (μg/d) - 75-90
- Ca (mg/d) - 1000-1300
- P (mg/d) - 700-1250

Generally, a pregnant woman requires about 60 g of protein daily (3 meat servings or equivalent) and 4 to 5 cups of milk (or equivalent). Diet should include 2 to 4 servings of fruit and 3 to 5 servings of vegetables. Simple carbohydrates (sugar, flour) should be limited and replaced by whole grains, which are high in B vitamins. Fat should constitute about 30% of total caloric intake.

Maternal malnutrition

Maternal malnutrition can have a profound effect on the developing fetus. If malnutrition occurs during the stages of cell division, then cells may not divide properly, causing permanent damage. If malnutrition occurs when cells are enlarging, then correcting the nutritional deficit can reverse damage. Recommendations for maternal weight gain:

- Underweight: 28-40 lb.
- Normal weight: 25-35 lb.
- Overweight: 15-25 lb.
- Obese: 15 lb.

Malnourished or underweight mothers have increased perinatal losses and preterm births. Neonates often have lower Apgar score and low birth weight (<2500 g). Women with eating disorders are more likely to have infants that are small for gestational age. Vitamin and mineral deficiencies can cause abnormalities in the developing fetus:

- Thiamine: Congestive heart failure, stillbirths.
- Folic acid: Megaloblastic anemia, neural tube defects.
- Vitamin D and calcium: Skeletal defects.

Infants of obese and morbidly obese women are often macrosomic (large) and may suffer fetal distress, early neonatal death, meconium aspiration, shoulder dystocia, and/or complications from Caesarean birth.

Folic acid

Folate/Folic acid is necessary for synthesis of DNA and RNA and cell duplication. Folic acid deficiency causes megaloblastic anemia in which immature red blood cells enlarge rather than divide, resulting in fewer red blood cells. Because of the need for cell duplication during pregnancy, adequate folic acid is critical, especially because there is increased urinary excretion and fetal uptake. Women should receive 0.4mg folic acid daily and, for deficiency, 1mg folic acid and iron supplements (because folic acid deficiency is associated with iron deficiency anemia). Deficiency may be difficult to diagnose because folate levels fluctuate with diet. Women with inadequate folic acid intake often exhibit nausea, vomiting, lack of appetite and low hemoglobin. Folic acid deficiency is associated with neural tube defects, such as myelomeningocele, spina bifida, and anencephaly, in the fetus.

Iron

Iron is necessary for the development of red blood cells. During pregnancy, the mother's plasma volume increases by about 50 percent, but red cell mass increases less, so the hematocrit drops from a normal of 38 to 47% to as low as 34% (physiologic anemia of pregnancy). Because the fetus takes iron from the mother, the mother's iron intake must compensate for this loss. Recommended daily iron supplements include the following:

- Hematocrit within normal range: 30 mg elemental iron daily
- Maternal iron deficiency anemia: 60 to 120 mg/daily until hematocrit normalizes, at which point the dose should decrease to 30 mg daily

When hemoglobin falls <11 g/dL, the mother is at increased risk of infection, pre-eclampsia, and postpartal hemorrhage with associated dangers to the fetus. If hemoglobin falls <6 g/dL, the mother may suffer cardiac failure, and the fetus is at high risk through increased rates of miscarriage and stillbirths, low birth rate, and neonatal death.

Fetal growth and development

Conception to 12 weeks

The stage of the embryo begins 15 days after conception. During this stage, organs begin to form, and external features become evident. The infant is most vulnerable to teratogenic agents during the time that organs are developing. The following is the development of embryo by week:

- Week 3 - The embryo elongates with a larger cephalic end than caudal. A long tube is developing for the brain and spinal cord and another for the GI system. The primitive tubular heart is forming outside the body cavity of the embryo. Teratogens may cause congenital limb absence.
- Week 4 - The heart beats regularly, and arm, leg, and tail buds are evident. The primordia of the eyes and ears are beginning to form. Teratogens may cause omphalocele, tracheoesophageal fistula, or hemivertebrae.
- Week 5 - Eyes (laterally-positioned) and nasal pits are forming. The C-shaped body has a large head and tail. By the end of week 5, arm and leg buds with paddle-like hands and feet are evident. Teratogens may cause cataracts, microphthalmia, facial clefts, and/or carpal/pedal ablation.
- Week 6 - Arms and legs are growing and digits forming. The jaws, upper lip, palate, and ears are developing. The tail is receding. The heart has chambers and is pumping blood through the circulatory system. Teratogens may cause septal/aortic defects, cleft lip, and/or agnathia.
- Week 7 - The head is assuming a round shape, and eyes are moving closer together. The mouth is formed and tongue developing. Eyelids are forming. The GI and urinary tracts have separated. Fetal heartbeats are detectable. Teratogens may cause intraventricular septal defects, pulmonary stenosis, cleft palate, epicanthus, micrognathia, short head, and sexual ambiguity.
- Week 8 - The embryo is about 3 cm C-R (crown to rump) length and resembles a human being, but the gender is not yet identifiable. Long bones are beginning to form, the heart has developed, the circulatory system is established, and muscles contract. Nose, eyes, and ears are evident. Teratogens may cause persistent atrial septal opening and shortening of digits.
- Weeks 9-12 - After 8 weeks, the embryo is considered a fetus as all organs and external structures are present to some degree. After 9 weeks, the fetus has reached about 5 cm C-R in length and 14 g in weight with the head comprising about 50% of the total size. The neck is evident and separate from the trunk. At 12 weeks, the fetus has reached 8 cm C-R in length and 45 g in weight, and facial features are more developed. The fetus appears human with a nose, small chin, and ears. Lip movement (sucking) may be seen, and tooth buds appear. Limbs have lengthened, and digits are well formed with arms longer and more developed than the legs. The fetus can make a fist. The urinary system has developed, and differentiated genitals appear. The fetus has spontaneous movement, and fetal heart tones are heard by Doppler.
- Weeks 13-16 - At 13 weeks, the fetus has reached 9 cm C-R in length and 55-60 g in weight. Growth is rapid during this period, and the gender should become evident. Eyelids have formed and can blink, and lanugo develops. The skin is transparent, so vasculature shows through. Sweat glands and fingerprints (fingers and toes) begin to develop. Bones and muscles are growing and developing, and the fetus is much more active. The fetus makes sucking movements, swallows amniotic fluid, and

produces meconium. The bronchial tubes branch out, and the liver and pancreas begin to produce secretions. By week 16, the bones begin to ossify.

- Week 20 - At 20 weeks, the fetus is 19 cm C-R in length and 435 to 465 g in weight and is covered with lanugo with increased scalp hair. Brown fat deposits make skin more opaque, and nipples are evident. Nails, eyebrows, and eyelashes are forming. The muscles are more developed. The fetus can suck the thumb and yawn and is increasingly active, felt as quickening by the mother.
- Week 24 - At 24 weeks, the fetus measures 28 cm C-H (crown to heel) in length and weighs 780 g. The lungs are developing with alveoli forming. The eyes have formed completely. The grasp and startle reflexes are obvious by the end of 24 weeks. There is little subcutaneous fat, so the skin is wrinkled and reddish in color but is completely covered with vernix caseosa. The palms and soles of the feet have thickened, and skin ridges are evident. Hair, eyebrows, and eyelashes are growing. The fetus remains active, sometimes hiccoughing and responding to sounds and activity by moving.
- Weeks 25-28 - At 25 to 28 weeks, the brain and central nervous system are developing and regulating some body function. The eyelids open and close, and the lungs are developed enough to provide gas exchange. Testes begin to descend into the scrotum. By week 28, the fetus measures 35 to 38 cm C-H in length and weighs 1200 to 1250 g. The fetus may be viable if delivered prematurely but will require extended intensive care.
- Weeks 29-32 - By week 32, the fetus measures 38 to 43 cm C-H in length and weighs 2000 g with increased muscles and fat, so the skin is less wrinkled. The pupillary response is present. Lungs are still immature, but the central nervous system can control breathing and temperature. Bones are developed but soft. Testes may have descended.
- Weeks 35-36 - By week 36, the fetus has gained more subcutaneous fat, so the skin is smoother and shedding lanugo. The brain is well developed, and lungs are almost developed. The fetus measures 42 to 48 cm C-H in length and weighs 2500 to 2750 g. Nails have grown to the ends of the digits, and the hands can grasp. The fetus orients to light. If delivered, the neonate has a good chance of survival. Testes have descended to the upper scrotum for males, and the labia majora and labia minora are equal size for females.
- Week 38-40 - By week 38, the fetus is full-term, measuring about 48 to 52 cm C-H in length and weighing 3000 to 3600 g. Males tend to be slightly larger than females, but wide variations occur. The fetus is plumper with smooth skin, and lanugo remains primarily on the shoulders and upper arms with scalp hair about 1 inch in length. The head remains slightly larger than the chest, which is prominent with protruding mammary glands. Testes have fully descended or are palpable in the inguinal canals. The labia majora are well developed with the labia minora smaller or covered. By this time, amniotic fluid has decreased to about 500 mL as the fetus fills the uterus. The fetus gains protective antibodies from the mother. Vernix caseosa remains present, more obvious in skin folds and creases. The fetus usually has turned with the head pointed downward toward the birth canal. Delivery usually occurs around week 40.

Intrauterine growth restriction

When a fetus does not fulfill his or her growth potential for any reason, the diagnosis is intrauterine growth restriction (IUGR). Prenatal ultrasound is used to diagnose IUGR, which is associated with oligohydramnios (decreased amniotic fluid) and pre-eclampsia (pregnancy-induced hypertension and proteinuria). IUGR is classified as symmetric or asymmetric, based on the size of the newborn's head:

- Symmetric IUGR:
  - Both head and body are small (growth-restricted).
  - Occurs early in pregnancy.
  - Common causes are chromosomal abnormalities and infections.
- Asymmetric IUGR:
  - Large head in proportion to the body; the head is spared.
  - The head is normal in size for gestational age, while the body is growth-restricted.
  - Occurs late in pregnancy.
  - Common causes include placental insufficiency and preeclampsia.

Fetal macrosomia

Fetal macrosomia, an exceptionally large fetus, poses problems for vaginal delivery because of the size of the infant. Fetal macrosomia is defined variably as >90th percentile for weight according to gestational age or > 4500 g. Fundal height >4 cm above expected for gestational age may be an indication. Fetal macrosomia is common with infants of diabetic mothers as well as obese mothers or those who gain an excessive amount of weight during pregnancy. Complications include prolonged second stage of labor because of over-stretching of the myometrium. If the fetus is too large to descend, uterine rupture may occur. Vaginal birth often results in lacerations or extensive episiotomy. The mother has increased risk of post-partum hemorrhage. The most common complication is shoulder dystocia, sometimes resulting in permanent brachial plexus injury to the neonate. Identifying fetal macrosomia prior to labor helps to prevent complications, but ultrasound and palpation are not always reliable when estimating fetal size/weight.

Preparation for labor

Classes to prepare parents for pregnancy and labor

Pre-pregnancy & first trimester: Classes that focus on becoming pregnant or understanding the early stages of pregnancy often cover methods of ensuring a healthy pregnancy and preventing complications. Topics may include sexuality, nutrition, lifestyle changes, and exercise as well as fetal development and gestational changes.

Second and third trimester: Later classes focus more on the birth process and labor as well as the postpartum period. Infant stimulation techniques, such as stroking the abdomen, rocking, and playing music help to develop early parental bonding and skills. Topics covered may include discussions of birth choices (natural childbirth, epidural, spinal, C-section), episiotomy, and circumcision as well as discussions of safety measures, such as infant car seats and types of cribs.

Adolescent: Classes that focus on adolescent mothers help the young mothers adapt to changes in their bodies and cope with psychosocial changes as well as preparing them for labor and delivery.

Bradley method
The Bradley method of natural childbirth is usually taught in a series of 12 weekly classes in which the pregnant woman and her partner participate. Classes are small (3 to 6 couples), and the goal is for natural childbirth without the use of drugs, C-section, or episiotomy to ensure both the mother and infant are healthy. Classes begin with a focus on the woman's health, including avoiding risk factors, ensuring good nutrition, and learning to handle pain. All issues related to pregnancy, such as anatomy, physiology, fetal changes, sexual activity, and breastfeeding are discussed. The role of the father/coach and the importance of bonding exercises are stressed. The couple learns methods to help promote relaxation and control pain during all stages of labor and delivery, using breath control and deep abdominopelvic breathing. The couple also learns about the needs of the newborn and routine care.

Lamaze method
The Lamaze method encourages women to take control of their bodies and utilizes various techniques (dissociation relaxation, relaxation exercises, and breathing patterns) to alleviate discomfort and facilitate birth. Lamaze teaches that birth is a natural process that should be as free of interventions/ medications as possible. Birthing practices include the following:

- Natural onset of labor without induction is encouraged.
- Movement during labor—walking, rocking, sitting on a birth ball, taking a shower—rather than lying in bed is encouraged.
- A support system is suggested, including partner as well as a person knowledgeable about birth, such as a doula, midwife, or friend.
- Only necessary medical interventions are recommended: Food and drink should not be restricted. Methods to speed labor, such as artificial rupturing of membranes, should be avoided as well as continuous fetal heart monitoring because it restricts the mother's activities.
- Avoidance of supine delivery is recommended: The upright, side-lying, and hands and knees positions are taught for use during different phases to speed or slow labor. Directed breathing techniques are also taught.
- Skin-to-skin contact at birth and rooming-in are encouraged practices.

Kitzinger method
The Kitzinger (psychosexual) method encourages women to take an active part in the birthing process, which is viewed as very natural. Kitzinger encourages alternatives to the usual hospital birthing procedures, including home births, birth rooms, and water births. Women are taught chest breathing combined with abdominal relaxation, touch relaxation, and visualization. The Kitzinger method relies on sensory memories, using some acting techniques to help women get in touch with feelings as well as specific movements (called "birth dance") to use during labor to reduce discomfort. In addition, the Kitzinger method includes educating the mother about pregnancy (including both physical and emotional development), fetal development, options available to her, and social and cultural aspects of birth. Women are encouraged to create a birth plan.

HypnoBirthing Method
The HypnoBirthing method combines natural birthing and self-hypnosis to help the mother eliminate stress and fear related to birthing. The mother is taught methods to relax the

mind and body and encourage production of natural endorphins. HypnoBirthing includes teaching the mother different relaxation and breathing techniques (such as deep breathing and slow breathing), pushing techniques, and birth positions. The partner is taught to use therapeutic touch and prompts to help the mother. Additionally, HypnoBirthing includes general education about pregnancy (including early labor signs), nutrition, exercise, breastfeeding, and bonding as well as post partum depression. One characteristic technique is "breathing the baby down" by inhaling and then exhaling while visualizing the energy going toward the fetus while tilting the pelvis up and gently bearing down. While bearing down, the mother visualizes the vagina opening to allow passage of the fetus.

Braxton-Hicks contractions—"false labor" vs true labor

Braxton-Hicks contractions, also known as "false labor," occur during the third trimester with uterine contractions only. Uterine contractions occur throughout pregnancy but are often too mild for the woman to feel; however, as birth nears, the contractions become stronger and may be mistaken for true labor. Braxton-Hicks:

- Contractions remain short in duration.
- Contractions occur at irregular intervals, which do not shorten over time.
- Pain is typically felt in the lower abdomen.
- Activities (walking, taking a warm bath, resting, or drinking ample fluids) may relieve pain and lesson contractions.
- Mild analgesia may relieve discomfort.
- The cervix remains unchanged.

True labor contractions:

- Contractions begin short in duration, but duration increases.
- Contractions occur at regular intervals, which typically shorten over time and contractions become more frequent.
- Pain typically is felt first in lower back and then radiates anteriorly to the abdomen.
- Activities may cause an increase in pain and frequency and intensity of contractions.
- Mild analgesia usually does not provide pain relief.
- Cervical effacement and dilatation are evident.

Signs of impending labor

The following signs of impending labor usually occur between weeks 38-42:

- Lightening - As the fetal head engages and moves toward the birth canal, the fundal pressure on the diaphragm lessons, so the mother can breathe more easily, but pressure in the pelvic area increases, causing urinary frequency. The lower abdomen may protrude more than previously. Increased circulatory impairment may cause venous stasis and ankle edema. In addition, there may be increased vaginal secretions as vaginal mucous membranes become congested. Pressure on the nerves may result in leg cramps or increased pelvic and leg pain.
- Braxton-Hicks contractions - Intensity and frequency of B-H contractions often increase immediately prior to onset of true labor.
- Change in energy - Mothers often experience a burst of energy and exhibit "nesting" activities, such as organizing the infant's room, preparing food, and cleaning house, usually in the week before labor starts.
- Bloody show - A mucous plug from pooled secretions forms at the opening of the cervical canal during pregnancy, and when the cervix begins to efface, this mucous

plug is expelled, exposing capillary vessels that bleed. The bloody show typically appears as pink mucous as opposed to the more brownish discharge associated with manual vaginal examination of the cervix. Bloody show usually occurs within 24 to 48 hours of the onset of labor.

- Cervical changes - The cervix ripens (softens) to allow for effacement and dilation.
- GI upset - Some of the symptoms often associated with the first trimester of pregnancy may return as labor nears. These symptoms include nausea, vomiting, heartburn, and diarrhea.
- Pain - Relaxin hormone production increases markedly (10 X) during pregnancy to relax the pelvic joints and allow them to expand, but this may result in pain, especially in the lumbosacral and pelvic areas.
- Membrane rupture - Rupture of the membranes occurs in about 12% of women prior to the onset of labor, which usually then occurs within 24 hours. Before rupture, the membranes typically bulge through the dilating cervix, and fluid comes in a gush, although it may come in smaller spurts in some cases. If the membranes rupture before engagement of the fetal head, the umbilical cord may prolapse with the fluid, increasing risk to the fetus, so mothers should be advised to always seek medical attention after rupture. If the mother is term and labor does not start within 24 hours of rupture, labor may be induced.
- Weight loss - Estrogen and progesterone levels cause a change in fluid balance that often results in a 1 to 3 pound loss of weight prior to onset of labor.

The following are evaluation procedures to assess onset of labor:

- History - Records should be reviewed and the mother questioned about the onset of contractions, frequency, and duration, and whether membranes have ruptured or vaginal bleeding has occurred.
- Leopold maneuvers - Abdominal palpations are done to establish fetal position, including lie, presentation, and position. Four maneuvers include (1) determining which fetal part is at the fundus, (2) locating the fetal extremities, (3) identifying the presenting part (head, breech) of the fetus, and (4) palpating for cephalic prominence.
- Vaginal exam - Speculum exam should precede digital exam if it is unclear whether membranes have ruptured. Vaginal exam to check for effacement and dilation is usually delayed until after labor begins. The position of the cervix is checked: Anterior position usually indicates the fetus is descending and applying pressure.
- Fetal station - The level of the fetal presenting part is determined in relation to the ischial spines. Level with the ischial spines (indicating engagement) is designated as station 0 with levels above designated with minus (-) signs and below with plus (+) signs.

Common discomforts of pregnancy

The following are common discomforts of pregnancy:

- Heartburn
    - Cause - Increased progesterone combined with decreased GI motility, relaxation of the cardiac sphincter, and upward displacement of stomach from pressure of the growing uterus increase esophageal reflux.
    - Management - Eat 4-5 small meals rather than 3 large meals daily. Take low sodium antacids (NOT sodium bicarbonate). Avoid lying down within 2 hours of eating. Avoid fried or spicy foods that trigger symptoms.
- Ankle/foot edema
    - Cause - Increased sodium retention from hormonal changes, circulatory impairment to lower extremities from pressure of uterus during 2nd and 3rd trimesters, prolonged sitting/standing, and increased permeability of capillaries cause edema.
    - Management - Elevate feed and legs when sitting. Avoid restrictive clothing, socks, or other bands about legs. Exercise feet frequently while sitting. Walk to promote increased circulation.
- Ptyalism
    - Cause - The cause is unclear for bitter salivation during first trimester.
    - Management - Use astringent mouth-washes. Chew gum or suck on hard candy.
- Nasal stuffiness/Bleeding
    - Cause - Increased production of estrogen during the first trimester causes swelling and irritation of mucous membranes.
    - Management - Use cool-air vaporizer. DO NOT use nasal sprays/decongestants.
- Vaginal discharge/Monilial infection
    - Cause - Increased estrogen promotes hyperplasia of vaginal mucosa and increased production of mucous. Warm moist environment promotes Candida monilial infection.
    - Management - Bathe daily. Wear cotton panties (NOT nylon or pantyhose). AVOID douching, panty liners, and tight clothing. Topical treatments: Miconazole, butoconazole, clotrimazole, tioconazole, nystatin, or terconazole.
- Leg cramps
    - Cause - Calcium/phosphorus imbalance occurs; increased pressure on nerves or impaired lower peripheral circulation from growing uterus, general fatigue, and pointing toes and shortening muscles may cause cramps.
    - Management - Dorsiflex feet to stretch muscles. Modify diet to improve calcium/phosphorus balance. Apply heat to cramping muscles. Change position slowly.
- Constipation
    - Cause - Increased progesterone levels slow intestinal motility. Pressure on intestines from enlarging uterus, inadequate diet/fluid intake, lack of exercise, and iron supplements all slow motility.
    - Management - Increase fluids and fiber in diet. Use stool softeners, such as DSS. AVOID laxatives, which may increase constipation over time.

- Hemorrhoids
    - Cause - Constipation and pressure on hemorrhoidal veins from the growing uterus cause veins to dilate.
    - Management - Treat constipation. Apply ice packs. Take Sitz baths. Apply topical ointments, such as Preparation H® or cortisone ointment. Apply topical anesthetic agent.
- Urinary frequency
    - Cause - Pressure of the growing uterus on the bladder during the first and third trimesters increases the frequency of urination.
    - Management - Increase fluids in the daytime and decrease ONLY in the evening if nocturia is present. Urinate when the urge is felt.
- Varicose veins
    - Cause - Venous congestion from pressure of uterus and impaired circulation, increased weight, age, and hereditary factors contribute to varicosities.
    - Management - Elevate feet and legs frequently. Avoid prolonged standing, crossing legs, and wearing constrictive hosiery or clothing. Wear support hose.
- Backache
    - Cause - Increased hormone levels cause softening of cartilage and increased lumbo-sacral curvature. Muscle strain, fatigue, poor body mechanics, and the carrying of twins contribute to backache.
    - Management - Do the pelvic-tilt exercise. Utilize correct body mechanics. Avoid heavy lifting, reaching for things on high surfaces, and wearing high-heeled shoes. Adjust height of work surfaces. Apply heat to lower back. Use back support in chair/bed. Begin modified exercise program, such as swimming, beginning with stretching. Stand straight and avoid slumping.

<u>Nausea and vomiting</u>

Causes of nausea and vomiting during pregnancy are as follows:

- First trimester: HCG secretion of the blastocyst and changes in carbohydrate metabolism cause nausea.
- Second and third trimester: Pressure of the growing uterus displaces the stomach upward and the intestines laterally and downward. Gastric emptying and peristalsis slows, causing bloating and constipation. Smooth muscles relax (from elevated progesterone), resulting in gastric reflux and heartburn, which further aggravate nausea and can lead to vomiting.

Preventive measures include:

- Eat small frequent meals.
- Avoid fatty, spicy foods.
- Eat simple carbohydrate foods, such as saltine crackers.
- Drink herbal tea with sugar or ginger ale.

Medical treatment includes:

- Antacids: Calcium carbonate, magnesium hydroxide, or magnesium oxide
- Antihistamine/anticholinergic: Meclizine
- Antiemetics: Ondansetron, prochlorperazine, promethazine, metoclopramide, or trimethobenzamide

Hyperemesis gravidarum: About 60-80% of pregnant woman suffer from nausea and vomiting (NV), especially during the first trimester, but only about 2% suffer severe (sometimes intractable) nausea and vomiting, known as hyperemesis gravidarum (HG). Nausea and vomiting may be associated with numerous disorders, including cholelithiasis, pancreatitis, hepatitis, and ectopic pregnancy, especially if accompanied by abdominal pain. Diagnosis includes physical examination to rule out other disorders, CBC with serum electrolytes, BUN, creatinine, and urinalysis. Symptoms include:

- Severe (sometimes intractable) nausea and vomiting
- Weight loss
- Dehydration.
- Hypokalemia
- Ketonemia
- Ketonuria (indication of inadequate nutrition)

Treatment includes:

- Intravenous fluids with 5% glucose in normal saline or Ringer's lactate.
- Oral fluids after nausea and vomiting controlled
- Antiemetic drugs
    - Acute treatment for NV and HG: promethazine (Phenergan®), prochlorperazine (Compazine®), or chlorpromazine (Thorazine®)
    - Maintenance for NV: Doxylamine with pyridoxine (Unisom®), diphenhydramine (Benadryl®), or cisapride (Propulsid®)
    - Maintenance for HG: Metoclopramide (Reglan®), trimethobenzamide (Tigan®), or ondansetron (Zofran®)

Antepartal tests (Alpha-fetoprotein)

Alpha-fetoprotein (AFT) is a protein produced by the yolk sac for the first 6 weeks of gestation and then by the fetal liver. Cutoff levels have been established for each week of gestation, with peak levels at about week 15. The test is used primarily to detect neural tube defects (NTDs), which develop in the first trimester. AFT can be measured in amniotic fluid or maternal serum. Triple screening includes serum AFT level done in the second trimester, and a positive result (which may be the result of errors in the duration of gestation) is followed by ultrasound and amniocentesis to check the amniotic AFT level. There is increased production of AFT with NTDs as well as abdominal wall defects and congenital nephrosis, so these levels can be used for assessment. (High quality ultrasound may also provide evidence of neural tube defects). The accuracy of tests varies depending upon the week of gestation. The most accurate results are acquired with testing during weeks 15-16.

Antepartal tests

Chorionic villus sampling

Chorionic villus sampling (CVS) in which a small sample of chorionic villi is obtained from the placenta can be done within the first trimester (≥10 weeks) to test for genetic/DNA and metabolic abnormalities, although CVS cannot detect neural tube disorders. The risk of miscarriage related to the procedure is now about the same as for amniocentesis (1: 1600); additionally, CVS can provide earlier diagnosis and fast results (within one day for some methods). For the procedure, an ultrasound is used to detect placental location, so the mother must drink fluids to fill the bladder. Sampling may be done transcervically with a catheter inserted through the cervix to the sampling site. Sampling may also be done transabdominally with local anesthesia and a needle inserted through the abdomen and uterine myometrium and advanced to the sampling site under ultrasound guidance.

PUBS

Percutaneous umbilical blood sampling (PUBS), also called cordocentesis, involves obtaining fetal blood from the umbilical cord in utero to diagnose hemophilias and other blood disorders, infection, and chromosomal abnormalities. During the procedure, an ultrasound is used to locate the umbilical cord and umbilical vein. A spinal needle is inserted through the abdominal wall and uterus and guided into the umbilical vein and a blood sample aspirated. A paralytic agent, such as pancuronium bromide, is often used to prevent the fetus from moving during the procedure. The mother must avoid deep breathing during the procedure as this may interfere with puncturing the vein. While any invasive procedure increases the risk of miscarriage, the rate of miscarriage with PUBS is only about 2%.

Amniocentesis

Amniocentesis is done at 15-20 weeks for genetic diagnoses and at 30-35 weeks to determine fetal lung maturity. Ultrasound locates the placenta and fetus and identifies an area with adequate amniotic fluid. The needle is inserted carefully to avoid major structures, the fetus, and arteries. A local anesthetic may be administered before insertion of a 22-gauge spinal needle into the uterine cavity. The first drops of fluid are discarded and a syringe attached. About 15-20 mL of amniotic fluid are withdrawn and placed in tubes, brown-tinted to shield the fluid from light that might break down bilirubin or other pigments. Ultrasound is again used to monitor removal of the needle, and the insertion point is checked for streaming (leakage of fluid). If the mother is Rh-negative, she is given Rh immune globulin immediately unless already sensitized. The fetal heart rate is monitored. Miscarriage occurs in about 1 in 1600. If performed at 11-14 weeks, there is increased risk to the fetus. Infection of the placenta (chorioamnionitis) is a rare complication.

Fetal lung maturity

Tests for fetal lung maturity are important for monitoring fetuses if there is an indication for early termination of pregnancy. Pulmonary maturity is often an important factor is neonatal survival as immaturity can result in respiratory distress syndrome (RDS). Tests of amniotic fluid include:

- Lecithin/sphingomyelin (L/S) ratio: The ratio of the phospholipids lecithin and sphingomyelin (two components of surfactant) changes during pregnancy with L/S ratio at 0.5:1 early in pregnancy, 1:1 at 30-32 weeks, and 2:1 at 35 weeks. At 2:1, RDS is unlikely, although this finding is not always accurate for infants of diabetic mothers (IDM), as they may show adequate ratio but still develop RDS; so these neonates must be monitored carefully. This test is not accurate if the amniotic fluid contains blood or meconium.
- Phosphatidylglycerol (PG): This phospholipid first appears in surfactant at about week 35 in IDM with complications and week 36 in other pregnancies. Its presence is a sign of lung maturity.

Commonly, both tests are done to confirm lung maturity.

Use of antepartal tests

Biophysical profile

Part 1: Fetal heart rate: Measures fetal heart rate and acceleration with movement as measured by the nonstress test (NST). The NST is done during the daytime with the woman in semi-Fowler's position with support under right hip to displace the uterus to the left. Two monitors are applied to the abdomen—an ultrasound transducer to measure FHR and a tocodynamometer to detect fetal movement. The monitoring continues for 20-40 minutes (time extended if fetus appears to be in sleeping cycle). Occasional decelerations are normal, but repeated decelerations correlate with increased risk of Caesarean section. The woman reports sensations of fetal movement and this is compared to recording of movement. Correlation of 50-90% is normal.

- Normal (Score 2): ≥ 2 FHR accelerations of 15 bmp above baseline for ≥ 15 seconds in a 20-40 minute period. (Reactive)
- Abnormal (0): 1-0 accelerations of FHR in 40 minutes. (Nonreactive)

Part 2: Respirations, movement, tone, amniotic fluid volume

- Fetal respirations - Assessed by ultrasound
    - Normal (Score 2) - ≥ 1 episode of rhythmic breathing for ≥30 seconds in a 30-minute period
    - Abnormal (0) - ≤30 seconds of rhythmic breathing in 30 minutes
- Fetal movement - Assessed by ultrasound and tocodynamometer
    - Normal (Score 2) - ≥ 3 separate movements in 30 minutes
    - Abnormal (0) - ≤2 movements in 30 minutes
- Fetal tone - Assessed by ultrasound
    - Normal (Score 2) - ≥ 2 episodes of extension and flexion of arm/leg (or opening/closing of a hand)
    - Abnormal (0) - No extension/flexion
- Amniotic fluid volume - Assessed by ultrasound and amniotic fluid index. Using the umbilicus as the point of reference, the abdomen is divided into 4 quadrants and the deepest pocket in each quadrant is measured. (The sum of 4 measurements equals the amniotic fluid index—AFI.)
    - Normal (Score 2) - At least one single vertical pocket >2 cm.
    - Abnormal (0) - Largest single vertical pocket is ≤2 cm.

Part 3: Scoring: The 5 different measurements for the biophysical profile are completed and scores (2 for normal and 0 for abnormal) are compiled and interpreted according to risk for asphyxia. Maximum score is 10:

- 10 - Normal fetus with no risk. No intervention indicated.
- 8 - Little/rare risk to fetus. No intervention indicated.
- 8 with abnormal amniotic fluid volume - Suspected chronic asphyxia. Increased risk of perinatal mortality ≤ 1 week (89:1000), so birth should be induced.
- 6 - Possible asphyxia. Induce birth if amniotic fluid volume abnormal, if fluid level is normal at >36 weeks with cervix favorable, and if repeat test is ≤6. Observe and repeat tests according to protocol if repeat test is >6.
- 4 - Probable asphyxia. Repeat test the same day to verify scores and induce birth if score ≤6.

- 2 - Asphyxia virtually certain. Marked increase in risk of perinatal mortality (125:1000), so birth should be induced.
- 0 - Certain asphyxia. Risk of perinatal mortality extremely high (600:1000), so birth should be induced.

Ultrasound

Ultrasound is an imaging technique using high-frequency sound waves to create computer images of vessels, tissues, and organs. Newer scans include 2-dimensional Doppler readings. Fetal ultrasound can be done at about the 5th week of gestation and is commonly done at 20 weeks for all pregnant women. Ultrasound may be done transvaginally or (more commonly) transabdominally to evaluate the gestational sac and embryo/fetus, providing the most accurate measurement of gestational age.

Purposes of ultrasound during the first trimester:

- Estimate gestational age (accuracy +/- 1-2 weeks).
- Assess vaginal bleeding.
- Determine multiple fetuses.
- Examine for indications of birth defects of the brain/spine.

Purposes of ultrasound during the second trimester:

- Estimate gestational age (accuracy +/- 2 weeks).
- Determine size and position of placenta, fetus, and umbilical cord.
- Examine for indications of major birth defects (cardiovascular/neural tube).

Purposes of ultrasound during the third trimester:

- Estimate gestational age (accuracy +/- 2-3 weeks).
- Assess fetal viability.
- Determine size and position of placenta, fetus, and umbilical cord.
- Estimate volume of amniotic fluid.

High-Risk Pregnancies

Pre-existing conditions

Gestational diabetes

American Diabetes Association Clinical Practice Recommendations for gestational diabetes include the following screening and diagnostic procedures:

- Assessment of risk should be done at initial visit and further testing for those at high risk: obese, previous GDM or delivery of infant >9 pounds, glycosuria, PCOS, or family history of type 2 diabetes.
- All women except those at very low risk should be tested at 14-28 weeks of gestation with one of two methods:
    1. Plasma/serum glucose 1 hour after 50-g glucose load with >140 mg/dL (threshold) diagnosing 80% of those with GDM. Those who exceed this threshold level should have a 100-g OGTT on another day.
    2. 100-g OGTT in the AM after 8-hour fast with TWO of the following fasting glucose levels diagnostic of GMS: Fasting ≥95 mg/dL; 1 hour ≥180 mg/dL; 2 hour ≥155 mg/dL; 3 hour >140mg /dL.

Very low risk women are <25 years with normal weight, no family or abnormal glucose history, no poor obstetrical outcomes or membership in high-risk ethnic group.

American Diabetes Association Clinical Practice Recommendations for diagnosis
The American Diabetes Association Clinical Practice Recommendations outline the 4 diagnostic categories of diabetes mellitus:

- Type I with insulin deficiency caused by destruction of β cells.
- Type 2 with insulin resistance and progressive defect in insulin secretion.
- Gestational occurring during pregnancy.
- Other types, such as genetic defect, pancreatic disease, or drug-induced.

Criteria for diagnosis of diabetes include ONE of the following:

- Fasting blood sugar ≥126 mg/dL after 8 hours of fasting. (The Hemoglobin A1C and 75-g oral glucose tolerance test [OGTT] are not recommended for initial diagnosis although A1C should be done on diagnosis and every 3 months to monitor average glucose level.)
- Hyperglycemic symptoms (polyuria, polydipsia, weight loss, blurred vision) with non-fasting plasma glucose ≥200 mg/dL. If symptoms are not equivocal, the test should be repeated on another day.
- Two-hour plasma glucose ≥200 mg/dL during a 75-g OGTT.

Criteria for pre-diabetes include:

- Impaired fasting glucose: 100-125 mg/dL.
- Impaired glucose tolerance: 2-hour plasma glucose of 140-199 mg/dL.

Pre-existing medical conditions

Diabetes mellitus
About 2% of women have or develop diabetes mellitus during pregnancy. Factors that affect maternal health include change in dietary habit (such as inadequate intake because of nausea and diarrhea), changes in hormones that affect glucose metabolism, and increased renal blood flow that interferes with tubular reabsorption and results in increased glucosuria. All of these factors make control of diabetes more difficult. Mothers are at increased risk of diabetic ketoacidosis, pregnancy-induced hypertension (preeclampsia), and diabetic retinopathy. Polyhydramnios (>2000 mL amniotic fluid) occurs in about 10%, increasing the risk of abruptio placentae, premature labor, and postpartal uterine atony. The risk of spontaneous abortion increases markedly if glucose levels are poorly controlled. Urinary tract infections, including pyelonephritis, may occur. Patient education is important to help the mother maintain adequate control of glucose with fasting AM plasma glucose at 90 to 100mg/100 mL and <120 to 140 mg/100 mL during the day. Diet recommendations include 35 kilocalories per kg of ideal body weight. Induction at week 38 or 39 is common.

Classes I-IV cardiac disease
The NY Heart association classifies heart disease by the functional capacity, and the maternal classification affects the fetus:

I. No cardiac insufficiency or activity limitations.
II. Slight activity limitations with symptoms present with ordinary physical activity.
III. Marked activity limitations with mild activity causing symptoms.
IV. Inability to carry out physical activities without severe symptoms.

There is minimal danger to the fetus for mothers in class I or II but increased risk to both the mother and the fetus for classes III and IV. Most mediations cross the placenta and the degree of safety during pregnancy has not always been established although most common drugs (heparin, digitalis glycosides, antiarrhythmics, thiazide and loop diuretics) are not teratogenic. For classes III and IV, delivery may be facilitated by low forceps or vacuum assistance, and Caesarean may be done if mother or fetus is in danger. Labor and delivery are particularly dangerous to the fetus because of inadequate oxygen and blood supply, so continuous fetal monitoring is essential.

Cardiopulmonary defects

With improved techniques of surgical repair of congenital heart defects, many women survive to childbearing age. Common maternal defects include tetralogy of Fallot, ventricular and atrial septal defects, patent ductus arteriosus, and coarctation of aorta. If surgical correction was successful, there is no added fetal risk, but if the condition was not completely repaired or involves cyanosis, pregnancy can put the fetus at risk because of inadequate oxygen supply (and 2-4% risk that the child will inherit the condition). Marfan's syndrome poses severe risks to the mother with mortality rates of 25-50% because of possible rupture of the aorta—also putting the fetus at risk. Additionally, because this is an autosomal dominant disorder, there is a 50% chance an infant will inherit. Mitral valve prolapse usually does not pose a risk to the fetus. Severe maternal cardiopulmonary disorders can result in death of the mother and/or fetus. However, the most common fetal complications are premature labor/birth and small for gestational age.

HIV/AIDS

Women with HIV/AIDS taking anti-retroviral drugs before conception should continue with the medications, although efavirenz is contraindicated because of teratogenic effects. If diagnosis occurs during the first trimester, then treatment should begin at that point or at the beginning of the second trimester. With treatment during pregnancy, the transmission rate from mother to fetus is about 2 percent. Usual treatment is 500-600 mg zidovudine (ZDV) in 2-5 doses daily from week 14. Caesarean delivery poses less chance of HIV transmission for the neonate but increases the risk of maternal infection. C-section is recommended if the mother lacked adequate prenatal care, the viral load is unclear or >1000 copies per mL at 36 weeks, or the mother had not received anti-retroviral drugs or had taken only ZDV or azidothymidine (AZT) during her pregnancy. IV ZDV is started 3 hours prior to C-section and used continuously through labor and delivery for vaginal delivery. HIV increases risk of maternal and fetal infections.

Maternal age

Adolescent

Adolescent mothers >15 are not at higher risk than those >20 if they have adequate prenatal care and follow guidelines and recommendations, but this is often not the case. Teenage mothers are more likely to smoke and to gain inadequate weight, increasing the likelihood of premature delivery, low-birth weight infants, iron deficiency anemia, and preeclampsia/eclampsia. Additionally, there is increased risk of cephalopelvic disproportion because the mother may not be fully matured physically. Teenagers (15-19) also have increased risk of sexually transmitted diseases (such as gonorrhea, herpes, chlamydia, and syphilis). Many also drink alcohol and take illicit drugs, increasing the incidence of fetal abnormalities. In many cases, the male partner is >20 and has little education, lacks employment, and may not be able to provide emotional or financial support. Adolescent partners are usually of similar social and educational background as the mothers and have not completed development and are not prepared for fatherhood. The nurse should remain non-judgmental and supportive, educating the adolescent and encouraging good prenatal care.

The following are common age-related adolescent responses to discovering pregnancy:

- Age ≤14 - Pregnancy may result from abuse, incest, or casual relationships, so the young mother rarely has a supportive partner. The girl is usually dependent of the parents, especially the mother who often makes the decisions. The girl may be very self-conscious about body changes, lack self-esteem, and have little knowledge about physiology or pregnancy.
- Age 15-17 - Pregnancy is more likely to result from an intimate relationship, but concern about peer or parental rejection is heightened. The mother is usually more knowledgeable about pregnancy and options (OTC pregnancy test, adoption, abortion) and may confirm pregnancy before confiding in others. The young mother and parents may differ in values related to terminating pregnancy/adoption.
- Age 18-19 - This young mother is more likely to confirm pregnancy early and on her own with an OTC pregnancy kit and has a better understanding of the consequences of pregnancy. Decisions about pregnancy depend on relationship with and support of partner and parents.

The following are adolescent responses to issues of pregnancy:

- First trimester - Confirmation of pregnancy is often delayed because of lack of awareness, denial, or fear. Physical changes (increased breast size) may cause embarrassment. The family (if told) may be angry, upset, unsupportive, and/or may pressure the mother to make a decision regarding abortion (pro or con).
- Second trimester - Changes in the body and quickening make it difficult for the teenager to ignore or deny pregnancy, but some try to hide pregnancy by wearing constrictive or baggy clothing and by dieting to retain pre-pregnancy weight. Family conflicts may arise as the family members learn about the pregnancy. The teenager may experience increased dependency and consider her own needs rather than the needs of the fetus.
- Third trimester - The teenager may be eager to get the pregnancy over with and is often fearful of or has nightmares about labor and delivery. Some may have trouble viewing the fetus as a separate being. Some, however, begin to prepare for childbirth by buying clothes or supplies for the baby.

<u>Mature, over 35</u>

Many women have chosen to delay pregnancy, resulting in a marked increase in pregnant women >35. These mothers tend to be better educated and more financially secure than younger mothers. If the mother is in good health, pregnancy poses little increased risk; however, the risk of death associated with pregnancy does increase with age. Those >40 have about 5 times the risk as those ≤24. Additionally, those >35 are more likely to have preexisting health problems, such as diabetes or hypertension, which increase risk. They are more likely to have a C-section, placenta previa, abruptio placentae, and spontaneous abortion. There may also be increased risk to the fetus. The incidence of Down syndrome increases with mothers >35 and more markedly >40, so these mothers are more likely to want genetic testing. Macrosomia and congenital malformations are also more common.

Older mothers with unplanned pregnancies may be concerned about their age, long-term care of the child, retirement plans, and lifestyle changes.

Multiple gestations

In vitro fertilization and ovulation-inducing drugs have increased the incidence of high order multiple gestations over the past 30 years. The trend of delayed childbearing has led to an increase in twin/multiple gestations. Infants born from multiple gestations are more likely to be born prematurely and with low birth weights. The incidence of premature birth and low birth weight is proportional to the number of fetuses. There may be growth restriction/growth discordance, oligohydramnios, and restriction of movement of one or more fetuses Approximately 50% of twins and 90% of triplets are born premature, compared to 10% of singletons. With this increase in prematurity and proportion of infants born with low birth weight, there are increased morbidities, such as cerebral palsy and intellectual disability. The risk for genetic disorders, such as neural tube defects, GI, and cardiac abnormalities, is twice that of single gestations.

Grand multiparity

Grand multiparity is ≥5 deliveries of live or stillborn infants at ≥20 weeks gestation; some studies suggest risks increase after 4 deliveries. Great grand multiparity is usually considered ≥10 deliveries. Risks associated with multiparity include increased incidence of placenta previa, abruptio placentae, preeclampsia, and hemorrhage. Rates of C-sections are increased significantly. Grand multiparas often have poor prenatal care and tend to have increased rates of disease, such as diabetes mellitus and hypertension, but studies show that with proper prenatal care, those without health problems have risks comparable to those with lower parity. Younger multiparous women have fewer complications than older multiparous women, so some of the increased risks may be primarily age-related. Fetal complications include macrosomia, SGA, and malpresentation (breech).

Infertility

Female infertility

The following are causes of female infertility:

- Non-patent fallopian tubes - Fallopian tubes may be scarred by PID, endometriosis, or adhesions. Tests are hysterosalpingography and laparoscopy.
- Ovulation failure - Hormone levels may be inadequate to promote ovulation. Ovarian cysts may interfere with ovulation. Testing includes checking hormone levels of luteinizing hormone and progesterone, and prolactin ultrasound (transvaginal).
- Cervical obstruction or uterine abnormality - Excess production of mucous or narrowing of the cervical os may prevent sperm from entering the uterus. Thickening, abnormalities, or growths (fibroids, cysts) of the uterus may prevent implantation. Testing includes hysteroscopy, endometrial biopsy, post-coital test, and ultrasound (hysterosonogram).
- Other - Sometimes no cause is found. Infertility may be age-related, as fertility decreases up to 5% annually >30 and decreases even more markedly >40. Testing varies.

Male fertility tests

In up to 30 percent of infertility cases, the male is responsible, so male fertility testing should be done as part of fertility assessment:

- Urogenital history & examination - A history should review drug abuse, smoking, exercise, STDs, and sexual behaviors. The male is examined for physical abnormalities, such as varicocele, and the testes evaluated for size.
- Semen analysis - Usually two different semen samples, from different times, are examined. Two normal tests usually indicate the male is fertile. The sperm count is calculated and the sperm examined for size, shape, and motility.
- Hormone levels - Testosterone and other hormone levels may be evaluated, but abnormal hormone levels are associated with only about 3 percent of male infertility cases.
- Genetic testing - Testing may identify Klinefelter's syndrome (male with an extra X chromosome) or Y microdeletion (cause of aspermia).

Assisted reproduction methods

The following are methods for assisted reproduction:

- Assisted reproduction therapy (ART) with egg and/or sperm donation - Donor eggs or sperm are combined with the partner's eggs or sperm before in intrauterine insemination.
- Gamete intrafallopian transfer (GIFT) - Sperm and ovum (gametes) are harvested/collected and inserted next to each other in the fallopian tube where normal fertilization takes place.
- Intracytoplasmic sperm injection (ICSI) - Individual harvested ovum is injected directly with individual sperm before intrauterine insemination. (May be part of ART)
- Intrauterine insemination (IUI) - Sperm are inserted directly into the uterus through a catheter. This procedure may follow hormone treatments to stimulate ovulation.
- In vitro fertilization (IVF) - Fertilized ova are inserted into the uterus, often after the woman takes drugs to stimulate production of ova and harvesting. Both or either ova or sperm may be donated.
- Zygote intrafallopian transfer (ZIFT) - Sperm and ova are combined and fertilization occurs outside the body, and then the zygotes are inserted into the fallopian tube where they travel to the uterus to implant.

Gonadotropins

Gonadotropin treatment requires administration of natural or recombinant hormones: follicle stimulating hormone (FSH) and luteinizing hormone (LH). Drugs include human chorionic gonadotropin (hCG), human menopausal gonadotropin (hMG) and recombinant human FSH (rFSH):

- Females who are not ovulating usually receive injections of hCG or hMG for 12 days to stimulate maturity of follicles and then one dose of hCG to trigger ovulation. About 60 percent become pregnant, but over half result in miscarriage. There is increased risk of multiple gestations, and ovarian enlargement or ovarian hyperstimulation syndrome may occur. Gonadotropins may also be used prior to harvesting of ova. Frequent ultrasounds and hormone levels are required to monitor the development of follicles.

- Males with low testosterone levels usually receive injections of hCG 3 times weekly for 4 to 6 months until testosterone levels increase. Then, men continue to receive injections of hCG or hMG 2 times weekly until sperm count is adequate. Gynecomastia may occur.

Fertility drugs

Bromocriptine reduces prolactin levels. Increased prolactin levels can interfere with ovulation in females and decrease testosterone levels and sperm production in males, resulting in impotence or erectile dysfunction. This drug is taken vaginally or orally 1 to 4 times daily, increasing the dose slowly to minimize side effects, which include headaches, dizziness, and GI disturbances. Clomiphene stimulates hormone production and ovulation in women whose estrogen levels and pituitary function are normal. Clomiphene is taken orally for 5 days during menstruation for 3 to 6 months with dosage adjusted according to results of Clomiphene challenge test (FSH levels). Males may take clomiphene to increase sperm counts. Clomiphene is often used to stimulate production of multiple ova prior to harvesting. Cabergoline actions are the same as bromocriptine, but cabergoline is only taken 1 to 2 times a week. Side effects are milder than bromocriptine, usually only headache. Gonadotropin-releasing hormone (GnRH) is administered prior to gonadotropin treatment to prevent pituitary from stimulating production of FSH and LH so production can be controlled.

Sexually transmitted disease

Cytomegalovirus

Cytomegalovirus, a member of the herpes simplex virus group, can cause asymptomatic infection in women. Over 50% of women are seropositive and may have chronic infections that persist for years. Cytomegalovirus is the most common intrauterine viral infection. Cytomegalovirus can be transmitted placentally or cervically during delivery (infecting ≤2.5% of neonates) and can put the fetus at high risk with death rates of 20-30% among infants born with symptoms. About 90% of survivors have neurological disorders, such as microcephaly, hydrocephalus, cerebral palsy, and/or intellectual disability. In less severe infections, symptoms (intellectual disability, hearing deficits, learning disabilities) may be delayed. Commonly, the neonate is small for gestational age (SVA). The brain and liver are commonly affected, but all organs can be infected. Multiple blood abnormalities can occur: anemia, hyperbilirubinemia, thrombocytopenia, and hepatosplenomegaly.

Herpes simplex virus

Most pregnant women infected with herpes simplex virus (HSV), usually type 2, are asymptomatic and unaware of infection. Most vertical transmissions occur when the neonate travels through a colonized birth canal. The risk of transmitting HSV during the birth process varies greatly, depending if the infection is a new infection (primary) or a secondary outbreak. The transmission rate from women with a primary HSV infection is approximately 50%, while the transmission rate is 1-2% if the infection is a recurrence of HSV. Signs of a neonatal infection with HSV include:

- Skin, eye, and mucous membrane blistering at 10—12 days of life.
- Disseminated disease may spread to multiple organs, leading to pneumonitis, hepatitis, and intravascular coagulation.
- Encephalitis may be the only presentation, with signs of lethargy, irritability, poor feeding, and seizures.

A mother with active herpes should deliver by Caesarean section within 4-6 hours after membranes rupture. An infant that is inadvertently exposed to an active lesion should be treated with acyclovir.

Chlamydia

Chlamydia is the most common sexually-transmitted disease in the United States and can be passed on at the time of birth if the infant is delivered vaginally and comes into contact with contaminated vaginal secretions. The organism responsible for this infection is *Chlamydia trachomatis.* Because the mother infected with this organism is usually asymptomatic, preventative care for the newborn is essential. The usual infection site for the newborn is the eye in the form of conjunctivitis. States now require all newborns be given a prophylactic dose of either erythromycin or tetracycline ointment in the eyes at birth to prevent this infection. While the antibiotic ointment stops the eye infection, a few infants exposed to the pathogen will develop pneumonitis and/or ear infection.

Syphilis

An infant can be exposed to the syphilis organism, *Treponema pallidum,* during gestation and become infected in utero starting with weeks 10-15 of gestation. Many infected fetuses abort spontaneously or are stillborn. The infant born infected with syphilis can be asymptomatic at birth or can have a full multi-system infection. An infant who is symptomatic may have non-viral hepatitis with jaundice, hepatosplenomegaly, pseudoparalysis, pneumonitis, bone marrow failure, myocarditis, meningitis, anemia, edema associated with nephritic syndrome, and a rash on the palms of the hands and soles of the feet. Other symptoms, such as interstitial keratitis and dental and facial abnormalities may occur as the child develops. Treatment involves an aggressive regimen of penicillin administration with frequent follow-up until blood tests are negative.

Neisseria gonorrhoeae

Neisseria gonorrhoeae infections are common and may result in recurrent infection, pelvic inflammatory disease (PID), chronic pain, and infertility. Women who become pregnant and have a history of gonorrhea with salpingitis are 7 to 10 times more likely to have an ectopic pregnancy. Signs of infection (dysuria and green foul-smelling discharge from the urethra and the vagina) may occur 3 to 5 days after contact. However, many women are asymptomatic, especially on initial infection. About 15% of those infected develop PID, sometimes requiring hospitalization. Those with suspected or confirmed infections must be treated aggressively with a broad-spectrum antibiotic with follow-up cultures 3 to 5 days after completion of therapy. Women who have multiple sex partners or use illicit drugs are at increased risk of gonorr*hea. Vaginal delivery increases risk to the neonate and can result in severe conjunctivitis, rupture of the globe, and blindness; however, routine prophylaxis (usually erythromycin ointment) to the neonate's eyes is effective treatment.

Human papillomavirus

Human papilloma virus (HPV) comprises >100 viruses. About 40 are sexually transmitted and invade mucosal tissue, causing genital warts (condylomata). HPV infection causes changes in the mucosa, which can lead to cervical cancer. Most HPVs cause little or no overt symptoms, but infections are very common, especially in those 15-25. Over 99% of cervical cancers are caused by HPV and 70% are related to HPVs 16 and 18. The HPV vaccine, Gardasil®, protects against HPVs 6, 11 (which cause genital warts), 16, and 18 (which cause cancer). Protection is only conveyed if the female has not yet been infected with these strains. The vaccine is currently recommended for females ≤26 years of age. Active lesions are resistive to treatment during pregnancy. If lesions are extensive, Caesarean delivery is recommended to avoid tearing and the need for suturing tissues with lesions as well as to decrease transmission to the infant, who may develop laryngeal papillomata (although risk is small).

Substance abuse

Marijuana, phencyclidine [PCP], and MDMA [ecstasy]

Marijuana, phencyclidine (PCP), and methylenedioxymethamphetamine (MDMA or ecstasy) are popular "club" drugs that may be used by some women during pregnancy:

- Marijuana: This is often used along with alcohol and tobacco, so effects are difficult to assess, but there do not appear to be teratogenic effects; however, some studies report exposure can result in fine tremors, irritability, and prolonged startle response for the first 12 months after birth.
- PCP: One of the biggest problems with PCP is that mothers may have an overdose or psychotic response that can result in hypertension, hyperthermia, and coma, compromising the fetus.
- MDMA: Ecstasy is a popular club drug that is frequently used by teenagers and young adults. There is no clear evidence regarding effects on the fetus although some research suggests it may cause long-term impairments in learning.

Amphetamines

Amphetamines are a class of drugs that cause CNS stimulation. The most commonly abused amphetamine is methamphetamine. Maternal use of these substances causes hypertension and tachycardia, which can cause miscarriage, abruptio placentae, and premature delivery. Vasoconstriction affects placental vessels, decreasing circulation, nutrition, and oxygen to the fetus. Additionally, users often have depressed appetite and may have malnutrition. Methamphetamines can cross the placental barrier and cause fetal hypertension and prenatal strokes and damage to the heart and other organs. The neonate is commonly small for gestational age, often ≤ 5 pounds, full term but ≤10 percentile for weight, with shortened length and smaller head circumference. The neonate in withdrawal from maternal amphetamine use will suffer abnormal sleep patterns, often characterized by lethargy and excessive sleeping during the first few weeks, poor feeding, tremors, diaphoresis, miosis, frantic fist sucking, high-pitched crying, fever, excessive yawning, and hyperreflexia.

Cocaine/crack

Cocaine/crack (freebase cocaine) is a nonopioid substance that readily crosses the placenta through simple diffusion. One of the most potent properties of cocaine is the ability of it to act as a vasoconstrictor. When a mother uses cocaine, the blood supply to the placenta is severely compromised when the vessels constrict, compromising blood flow and resulting in growth retardation and hypoxia. Cocaine also causes a programmed cell death (known as apoptosis) in the heart muscle cells of the fetus, resulting in cardiac dysfunction for the fetus. Maternal cocaine use increases the risk of premature birth and causes serious consequences for the neonate after birth, including cerebral infarctions, nonduodenal intestinal atresia, anal atresia, NEC, defects of the limbs, and genitourinary defects. Cocaine stimulates the central nervous system by limiting the uptake of certain neurotransmitters norepinephrine, serotonin, and dopamine. Cocaine has a direct toxic effect on the fetal nervous system, so the infant will exhibit extreme irritability and tremors followed by sluggish, lethargic behavior.

Heroin

Heroin, an illegal opioid narcotic, is highly addictive. Users are at increased risk of HIV/AIDS from sharing needles as well as cellulitis, endocarditis, and abscesses. Pregnant users may experience poor nutrition, iron deficiency anemia, and preeclampsia-eclampsia all negatively affecting the fetus. Premature birth, early placental separation, and breech presentation are common. If the mother tries to stop using heroin, she may go into withdrawal, which can trigger premature labor, spontaneous abortion, or stillbirth. Symptoms of withdrawal usually start within 12 hours and include agitation, insomnia, increased sweating, and runny nose, progressing to gastrointestinal effects that include cramping, diarrhea, nausea, and vomiting. Pregnant women may be placed on a program of methadone maintenance under careful medical supervision as methadone, while posing less danger to the fetus, is also addictive. However, methadone may delay withdrawal symptoms and reduce cravings. Additionally, while neonates may exhibit jitteriness, fever, poor feeding, and vomiting after birth, the symptoms are usually transient.

Methadone

Methadone is commonly used to treat women who are addicted to heroin as it blocks withdrawal symptoms and drug craving, but methadone crosses the placental barrier and exposes the fetus to the drug. Many female heroin users are of reproductive age, and methadone is often administered to pregnant women to decrease dangers associated with heroin, such as fluctuating levels of drug and exposure to hepatitis and HIV from sharing of needles. Exposure to methadone may result in miscarriage, stillbirth, intrauterine growth restriction, fetal distress, and low birth rate although symptoms are usually less severe than with heroin. However, if the mother takes methadone along with other drugs, this can compound the adverse effects. Additionally, sudden withdrawal from methadone may cause preterm labor or death of the fetus, so methadone should be monitored carefully.

Alcohol, FAS

Maternal ingestion of alcohol may result in Fetal alcohol syndrome (FAS), a syndrome of birth defects. Despite campaigns to inform the public, women continue to drink during pregnancy, but no safe amount of alcohol ingestion has been determined, and pregnant women should be advised to abstain. FAS includes:

- Facial abnormalities: Hypoplastic (underdeveloped) maxilla, micrognathia (undersized jaw), hypoplastic philtrum (groove beneath the nose), short palpebral fissures (eye slits between upper and lower lids).
- Neurological deficits: May include microcephaly, intellectual disability, and motor delay, hearing deficits. Learning disorders may include problems with visual-spatial and verbal learning, attention disorders, delayed reaction times.
- Growth retardation: Prenatal growth deficit persists with slow growth after birth.
- Behavioral problems: Irritability and hyperactivity. Poor judgment in behavior may relate to deficit in executive functions.

Indication of brain damage without the associated physical abnormalities is referred to as alcohol-related neurodevelopmental disorder (ARND).

Tobacco/nicotine

Tobacco smoke contains many substances, such as nicotine and carcinogens, known to be detrimental to a person's health. When a pregnant woman smokes, her fetus is exposed to carbon monoxide, nicotine, and hydrogen cyanide, which all cross the placenta. Carbon monoxide displaces oxygen from hemoglobin, resulting in decreased oxygen delivery to the fetus. Exposure increases risk of miscarriage and perinatal death. Infants exposed *in utero* to tobacco may have the following problems:

- Decreased length, weight, and head circumference.
- Increased rates of congenital birth defects, such as cleft palate or lip, limb reduction defects, and urinary tract anomalies.
- Increased incidence of placenta previa, placental abruption, and preterm birth.

If smoking continues after delivery, these further detrimental effects may occur:

- Sudden infant death syndrome.
- Increased infant respiratory tract infections and childhood asthma.
- Behavioral problems in later childhood.

Pregnant women may benefit from smoking cessation programs and increased education about the danger to the fetus.

Termination of pregnancy

Surgical procedures

Termination of pregnancy may be done before the time of fetal viability (up to 24 weeks) but increasingly, state regulations are limiting access to late-term abortions. Surgical procedures are as follows:

- Vacuum aspiration – (4 to 10 weeks) This may be done manually or by machine, with a cervical dilator used first and then a cannula passed into the uterus to suction the tissue.
- Suction curettage – (6 to 14 weeks) This is similar to vacuum aspiration, but a looped curettage is inserted into the uterus after the tissue is suctioned to remove any remnants.
- Dilation and extraction – (14 to 24 weeks) The cervix is dilated, and the fetus extracted by instrument. This is usually followed by suctioning to remove remnants. This procedure is common during the second trimester.
- Intact dilation and extraction – (>18 weeks) This "partial birth abortion" usually follows induced labor and removes the intact fetus via the cervix, but it requires prior feticide (intraamniotic or intrafetal digoxin or potassium chloride) to prevent live birth.
- Hysterectomy/ hysterotomy – (12 to 24 weeks) This procedure is used only as a last resort (rare).

Medical procedures

Medical procedures for termination of pregnancy can be used during the first trimester. Because medication-induced abortion always involves cramping and heavy bleeding, supervision should be available in case hemorrhage occurs. Mifepristone is administered orally on day 1 to block action of progesterone and change endometrium, and then misoprostol is administered vaginally or buccally on day 2 or 3 (or within 8 hours if bleeding is occurring) to cause contractions to help expel the embryo/fetus. Medical examination to ensure abortion is complete is done after 7 days. Methotrexate injection is administered on day 1 to stop cell division and growth of the embryo. This is followed by misoprostol administered vaginally on day 6 or 7 with examination on day 8 to ensure abortion is complete. In some cases, misoprostol or mifepristone may be used alone. If abortion is incomplete after medication-induced abortion, then suction and curettage may be necessary to remove retained tissue.

Complications

Spontaneous abortion

Vaginal bleeding during the first trimester of pregnancy may indicate spontaneous abortion, ectopic pregnancy, gestational trophoblastic disease, or infection. All women of childbearing age with an intact uterus presenting with abdominal pain or vaginal bleeding should be assessed for pregnancy. Abortion classifications:

- Threatened: Vaginal bleeding during first half of pregnancy without cervical dilatation.
- Inevitable: Vaginal bleeding with cervical dilatation.
- Incomplete: Incomplete loss of products of conception, usually between 6-14 weeks.
- Complete: Complete loss of products of conception, before 20 weeks.
- Missed: Death of fetus before 20 weeks without loss of products of conception within 4 weeks.
- Septic: Infection with abortion.

Diagnostic tests include:

- Pelvic examination.
- Laboratory tests: CBC, Rh factor, antibody screen, urinalysis, quantitative serum β-hCG level
- Ultrasound to rule out ectopic pregnancy.

Treatment includes:

- Suctioning of vaginal vault with Yankauer suction tip with pathologic examination of tissue.
- Evacuation of uterus for incomplete abortion.
- RhoGAM (50-150μg) for bleeding in unsensitized Rh-negative women.

Ectopic pregnancy

Ectopic pregnancy occurs when the fertilized ovum implants outside the uterus in an ovary, fallopian tube (the most common site), peritoneal cavity, or cervix. Diagnostic studies include vaginal exam, pregnancy test, transvaginal sonography (TVS) to rule out intrauterine pregnancy, hCG titers (increase more slowly with ectopic pregnancy). Progesterone level >22 helps rule out ectopic pregnancy.

Early symptoms

- Indications of pregnancy: amenorrhea, breast tenderness, nausea and vomiting.
- Positive Chadwick's sign (blue discoloration of cervix)
- Positive Hegar's sign (softening of isthmus).
- Bleeding may be the first indication as hormones fluctuate.
- Hormone hCG present in blood and urine.

Symptoms of rupture

- One-sided or generalized abdominal pain.
- Decreased Hemoglobin and hematocrit.
- Hypotension with hemorrhage.
- Right shoulder pain because of irritation of the subdiaphragmatic phrenic nerve.

Treatment

- Methotrexate IM or IV if unruptured and ≤3.5 cm in size to inhibit growth and allow body to expel.
- Laparoscopic linear salpingostomy or salpingectomy.

Fetomaternal hemorrhage/transfusion

Fetomaternal hemorrhage (FMH) occurs in many pregnancies without any signs or symptoms. A small amount of fetal blood in the maternal circulation (1-2 ml) (fetomaternal transfusion) has no clinical significance. Massive FMH (blood loss greater than 30 ml) occurs in about 3 of every 1,000 pregnancies, and is a major cause of stillbirths. Neonates' blood volume ranges from 85-100 ml/kg, so 30 ml of blood loss represents 10-12% of the blood volume in a 3 kg neonate. Neonates may present with anemia. Risk factors for FMH include maternal trauma, placental abruption, placental tumors, third trimester amniocentesis, fetal hydrops, and twinning. One test used to diagnose the presence of FMH is the Kleihauer-Betke (KB) test, in which a sample of the mother's blood is examined for the presence of fetal hemoglobin. The KB test estimates the amount of hemorrhage that has taken place.

Abruptio placentae

With abruptio placentae, the placenta prematurely detaches, partially or completely, from the uterus. An Abruptio placenta is related to maternal hypertension and incidence increases with cocaine abuse. Partial detachment interferes with the functioning of the placenta, causing intrauterine growth retardation. Severe bleeding occurs with total detachment. Diagnosis includes ultrasound, CBC and type and cross match, and coagulation studies (50% have coagulopathy). Symptoms include:

- Vaginal bleeding.
- Tender uterus with increased resting tone.
- Uterine contractions (hypertonic or hyperactive.
- Nausea and vomiting (in some patients).
- Dizziness.
- Complications include fetal distress, hypotension and DIC, as well as fetal and/or maternal death.
- Fetal death common with ≥50% separation.
- Irreversible brain damage may occur with fetal hypoxia, and neurological deficits occur in about 14% of survivors.

Treatment includes:

- Gynecological consultation.
- Crystalloids to increase blood volume.
- Fresh frozen plasma for coagulopathy.
- Partial: Bedrest and monitoring.
- Complete: Immediate vaginal or C-section delivery.

Placenta previa

Placenta previa occurs when the placenta implants over or near the internal cervical os. Implantation may be complete (covering the entire opening), partial, or marginal (to the edge of the cervical opening). Women with placenta previa have increased incidences of hemorrhage in the third trimester. Symptoms include painless bleeding after 20th week of gestation. Diagnosis is per ultrasound. Vaginal examination with digit or speculum should be avoided. The condition may correct itself as the uterus expands, but bed rest may be needed. Emergency C-section is done for uncontrolled bleeding. In infants, placenta previa is associated with poor growth, anemia, and increased risk of congenital anomalies in their central nervous systems, heart, respiratory, and gastrointestinal tracts. Placenta previa may also cause premature birth with associated neonatal complications of prematurity.

Hypertensive disorders of pregnancy

Hypertensive disorders of pregnancy comprise a continuum ranging from mild to severe:

- Hypertension: BP >140/90 or 20-mm Hg increase in systolic or 10-mm diastolic. May be chronic or transient without signs of preeclampsia or eclampsia.
- Preeclampsia: Hypertension associated with proteinuria (300mg/24h) and edema (peripheral or generalized) or increase of ≥ 5 pounds of weight in one week after 20th week of gestation. Severe preeclampsia is BP ≥ 160/110. Symptoms include headache, abdominal pain, and visual disturbances.
- Eclampsia: Preeclampsia with seizures occurring at 20th week of gestation to 1 month after delivery.
- HELLP syndrome (hemolysis, elevated liver enzymes (AST and ALT), and low platelets (<100,000). Usually accompanied by epigastric or right upper quadrant pain.

Treatments include:

- Chronic hypertension: Methyldopa beginning with 250mg every 6 hours.
- Preeclampsia, eclampsia, HELLP:
  - Delivery of fetus (may be delayed with mild pre-eclampsia if < 37 weeks gestation)
  - Magnesium sulfate IV 4-6 g over 15 minutes initially and then 1-2 g per hour.
  - Antihypertensive drugs.

Pre-eclampsia and eclampsia

Pregnancy-induced hypertension (also called preeclampsia or toxemia) is a disorder that develops in approximately 5% of all pregnancies. Its main features are elevated blood pressure and proteinuria that develop around 20 weeks of gestation. Initial treatment of pre-eclampsia is magnesium sulfate to prevent seizures in the mother. Eclampsia occurs with seizures. Severe cases may require the premature delivery of the infant to relieve the condition. The main detrimental effect on the fetus occurs because of longstanding hypertension that leads to utero-placental vascular insufficiency, which impairs the transfer of nutrients and oxygen to the fetus, resulting in intrauterine growth retardation (IUGR). Placental abruption also occurs more frequently. The IUGR is usually asymmetric (fetal head size is normal for gestational age). Infants who are born with IUGR and/or prematurity have increased morbidity and mortality. Treatment includes antihypertensive medications, such as thiazide, hydralazine, propranolol, labetalol, nifedipine and methyldopa as well as anticonvulsants if seizures occur.

HELLP syndrome

HELLP syndrome occurs in 4 to 12% of those with pre-eclampsia, most often during weeks 27 to 37 but may develop within 24 hours post-partum, and is characterized by:

- H—hemolysis.
- EL—Elevated liver enzymes
- LP—low platelet count.

HELLP syndrome is most common in older multiparous mothers. Hypertension may be less pronounced than in others with preeclampsia. Pain in the right upper quadrant related to liver dysfunction may be misdiagnosed as gastrointestinal upset or gall bladder disease. Mothers often present with flu-like non-specific symptoms, including headache, nausea and vomiting and visual disturbances. Prompt diagnosis and treatment are necessary because of high mortality. Platelet transfusions are given if platelet counts $<20,000/mm^3$ or $<50,000$ mm^3 with Caesarean. The primary treatment is immediate delivery of the fetus as the mother may develop hepatic hemorrhage or permanent liver damage. Both the mother and the fetus are at risk. Neonates are at increased risk and may require mechanical ventilation. Complications include abruptio placentae, DIC, and post-partum hemorrhage.

DIC, pathology

Disseminated intravascular coagulation (DIC) (consumption coagulopathy) is a secondary disorder of pregnancy. DIC may be triggered by abruptio placentae, uterine rupture, embolism of amniotic fluid, eclampsia, post-partum hemorrhage, shock (hypovolemic), severe infection with sepsis, and saline/missed abortion. DIC triggers both coagulation and hemorrhage through a complex series of events that includes trauma that causes tissue factor (transmembrane glycoprotein) to enter the circulation and bind with coagulation factors, triggering the coagulation cascade. This stimulates thrombin to convert fibrinogen to fibrin, causing aggregation and destruction of platelets and forming clots that can be disseminated throughout the intravascular system. These clots increase in size as platelets adhere to the clots, causing blockage of both the microvascular systems and larger vessels, and this can result in ischemia and necrosis. Clot formation triggers fibrinolysis and plasmin to breakdown fibrin and fibrinogen, causing destruction of clotting factors, resulting in hemorrhage. Both processes, clotting and hemorrhage, continue at the same time, placing the patient at high risk for death, even with treatment.

DIC, symptoms and treatment

The onset of symptoms of DIC may be very rapid or a slower chronic progression from a disease. Those who develop the chronic manifestation of the disease usually have fewer acute symptoms and may slowly develop ecchymosis or bleeding wounds. Symptoms include:

- Bleeding from surgical or venous puncture sites.
- Evidence of GI bleeding with distention, bloody diarrhea.
- Hypotension and acute symptoms of shock.
- Petechiae and purpura with extensive bleeding into the tissues.
- Laboratory abnormalities:
    - Prolonged prothrombin and partial prothrombin times.
    - Decreased platelet counts and fragmented RBCs.
    - Decreased fibrinogen.

Treatment includes:

- Identifying and treating underlying cause.
- Replacement blood products, such as platelets and fresh frozen plasma.
- Anticoagulation therapy (heparin) to increase clotting time.
- Cryoprecipitate to increase fibrinogen levels.
- Coagulation inhibitors and coagulation factors.

DIC panel

Disseminated intravascular coagulation (DIC) panel includes a number of tests. Generally, test results that measure materials needed for clotting are decreased and those that measure clotting times are increased. Typical findings that indicate DIC include:

- Activated partial thromboplastin time (aPTT) - Increased time
- Prothrombin time - Findings vary, may be increased time (in 75%), normal time (25%), or shortened (25%).
- Partial thromboplastin time - Increased time (in 50-60%).
- Thrombin time - Increased.
- D-Dimer - Increased (usually more reliable than FSP): D-dimer is a specific polymer that results when fibrin breaks down, giving a marker to indicate the degree of fibrinolysis.
- Fibrinogen - Decreased.
- Platelets - <100,000.
- Fibrin split products (FSP) - Increased (in 75-100%). FSPs occur as more clots form and more breakdown of fibrinogen and fibrin occurs, interfering with blood coagulation by coating platelets and disrupting thrombin, and attaching to fibrinogen so stable clots can't form.
- Clotting factor assays (V, VI, VII, X, XIII) - Decreased.
- Antithrombin III - Decreased (in 90%).

Rh incompatibility

Rh incompatibility occurs if the mother is Rh- and the father is Rh+, putting their infant is at risk for hemolytic disease of the newborn (HDN) or Rh disease, (erythroblastosis fetalis). Sensitization can occur during abortion, abruptio placenta, amniocentesis, cesarean section, chorionic villus sampling, cordocentesis, delivery, ectopic pregnancy, and toxemia. To prevent erythroblastosis fetalis, women who are Rh- with an Rh+ mate receive the serum RhoGAM®, containing anti Rh+ antibodies. The purpose of the antibodies is to agglutinate any fetal red blood cells that pass over into the mother's circulatory system and thus prevent the mother from forming antibodies against them that will attack the infant and sensitize her for future pregnancies.

- Mother receives 300 Φg RhoGAM (Rhlg, Rh immunoglobulin) intramuscularly at 26 to 28 weeks of pregnancy and again within 72 hours after her delivery.
- Miscarriage, ectopic, abortion: At ≤12 weeks, the mother receives50 Φg of MICRhoGAM®. At ≥13 weeks, the mother receives RhoGAM® as for pregnancy.

ABO incompatibility is similar but usually less severe although some infants require phototherapy for jaundice and/or exchange transfusion.

CHEAP TORCHES and TORCH panel

CHEAP TORCHES is the acronym used to recall common causes of congenital and neonatal infections. Many congenital infections are present for at least a month prior to birth and remain present at birth:

- C - Chickenpox (varicella)
- H - Hepatitis (B, C, & E)
- E - Enterovirus (RNA viruses, including coxsackievirus, echovirus, and poliovirus)
- A - AIDS (HIV)
- P - Parvovirus (B 19)
- T – Toxoplasmosis
- - Other (Group B streptococcus, Candida, Listeria, TB, lymphocytic choriomeningitis)
- R - Rubella (measles)
- C – Cytomegalovirus
- H - Herpes simplex virus
- E - Every other STD (Chlamydia, gonorrhea, Ureaplasma, papillomavirus
- S - Syphilis

Exposure to these pathogens *in utero* may cause a miscarriage or congenital defect, especially if the exposure was during the first trimester. Symptoms may include small for gestational age, enlarged liver and spleen, thrombocytopenia, skin rash, jaundice, seizures, or encephalitis. The "TORCH" panel, which tests for toxoplasmosis, rubella, cytomegalovirus, and herpes simplex virus, is commonly used to screen pregnant women for infectious diseases.

Terms associated with pregnancy

Gravida — Any pregnancy (including present) regardless of duration/outcome

Nulligravida — A woman who has never been pregnant

Primigravida — A woman with her first pregnancy

Multigravida — A woman in her ≥2nd pregnancy

Para — Delivery of live or stillborn fetus/neonate >20 weeks gestation

Nullipara — Woman who has not given birth >20 weeks gestation

Primipara — A woman who has given birth, live or stillborn, one time >20 weeks gestation

Multipara — A woman who has given birth, live or stillborn, ≥2 times >20 weeks gestation

Grand multipara — A woman who has given birth, live or stillborn, ≥5 times >20 weeks gestation

Term — 38 to 48 weeks duration of pregnancy

Gestation — Number of weeks since the first day of last menstrual period (LMP)>

Abortion — Death of fetus <20 weeks' gestation

Stillbirth — Death of fetus >20 weeks' gestation

Complications of Labor

Premature labor

Polyhydramnios

Polyhydramnios is increased amounts of amniotic fluid (>500 mL) present during fetal development and is associated with an elevated perinatal mortality rate. Approximately 25% of pregnant women with polyhydramnios experience preterm labor and delivery of a premature infant. Approximately 20% of infants born to mothers with polyhydramnios have an associated anomaly. Some conditions associated with polyhydramnios include:

- Obstructional lesions in the GI tract, such as duodenal atresia or tracheoesophageal fistula with esophageal atresia.
- Anencephaly.
- Central nervous system anomalies that impair the swallowing reflex.
- Cardiovascular rhythm anomalies associated with hydrops.
- Twin-twin transfusion syndrome in multiple pregnancies.
- Macrosomia.
- Fetal or neonatal hydrops.
- Chromosomal abnormalities such as trisomy 21, 18, or 13.
- Skeletal malformations such as congenital hip dislocation, clubfoot, or limb reduction.
- Increased risk for prolapsed umbilical cord and placental abruption.

Precipitous/precipitate labor

Precipitous/precipitate labor and birth occurs when onset of labor to birth takes only ≤3 hours, often because of strong uterine contractions and low muscle resistance in maternal tissue that promotes rapid dilation of the cervix (or lacerations) and descent of the fetus. A primigravida may dilate 5 cm per hour; and a multigravida, 10 cm per hour. The neonate may have a low Apgar score and is at increased risk for aspiration of meconium and intracranial injury, such as subdural/dural tears. The strong uterine contractions may interfere with uterine blood flow and oxygenation of the fetus. Precipitous birth alone (without obvious labor), by contrast, is usually an unexpected and sudden birth that takes place outside of the hospital or is unattended by a physician because there is no time to travel or get help. In these cases, the neonate is sometimes expelled into a toilet or onto the floor, causing injury.

Emergency birth

Prolapsed umbilical cord

A prolapse of the umbilical cord occurs when the umbilical cord precedes the fetus in the birth canal and becomes entrapped by the descending fetus. An occult cord prolapse occurs when the umbilical cord is beside or just ahead of the fetal head. About half of prolapses occur in the second stage of labor and relate to premature delivery, multiple gestation, polyhydramnios, breech delivery, and an excessively long umbilical cord. Some cases are precipitated by obstetric interventions, such as amniotomy, external eversion, and application of scalp electrode for monitoring. As contractions occur and the head descends, this applies pressure to the umbilical cord, occluding blood flow and causing hypoxia and bradycardia. The decrease in blood flow through the umbilical vessels can cause impaired gas exchange, and if pressure on the cord is not relieved, the fetus can suffer severe neurological damage or death. Management includes elevating the presenting part off the cord, having the mother elevate her knees to the chest, and preparing for C-section.

PROM, SROM, PPROM, and prolonged PROMO

Premature rupture of membranes (PROM): The amniotic sac breaks, ideally at term (40 weeks), prior to onset of labor. PROM occurs is labor fails to commence within an hour. About 80% go into labor within 24 hours, and if labor doesn't commence in 12-24 hours, the patient must be frequently monitored until labor begins to ensure adequate amniotic fluid remains, or labor may be induced to prevent infection if the child is at term. Spontaneous rupture (SROM) usually occurs in the early stage of labor during an intense contraction, causing the fluid to gush out the vagina.

Preterm premature rupture of membranes (PPROM) occurs in a woman <37 weeks of gestation and prior to the onset of labor. The patient is monitored as with premature rupture. It is one of the leading causes of premature birth.

Prolonged rupture of membranes: Prolonged PROM that persists for greater than 18-24 hours prior to the onset of labor. It is associated with increased risk of infection in the neonate.

Postterm pregnancy

Postterm pregnancy (>294 days or 42 weeks past 1st day of last menstrual period) occurs in 3-7% of pregnancies, and is often the result of errors in calculating due date, but true postterm pregnancies, while posing little risk to the mother, can increase risk to the fetus, and vaginal birth may be facilitated by forceps or vacuum extractor. Increased fetal risks include:

- Large for gestational age (LGA), >4500g (about 10 pounds), which may result in prolonged labor, birth trauma with fractures or neurological injury, or Caesarean section.
- Aspiration of meconium occurs more frequently because a large fetus is more likely to expel meconium.
- Post-maturity syndrome related to restriction of growth in the uterus, often because of restricted blood flow, putting the fetus at risk for respiratory and neurological disorders.

Oligohydramnios

Oligohydramnios is decreased amounts of amniotic fluid (<500mL). Amniotic fluid cushions the fetus during development and is also necessary for normal development of the lungs. After 20 weeks of gestation, amniotic fluid is mainly produced by the fetus' excretion of urine. Fluids secreted by the respiratory tract and the oral/nasal cavity also contribute to the production of amniotic fluid. Oligohydramnios signals significant congenital pathology in the fetus and is associated with an elevated perinatal mortality rate. Some conditions associated with oligohydramnios include:

- Urinary tract anomalies:
  - Obstructive uropathy.
  - Renal agenesis.
  - Polycystic kidneys.
- Pulmonary hypoplasia.
- Pressure deformities, such as clubbed feet.
- Compression of the umbilical cord, leading to fetal hypoxia.
- Meconium staining.
- Post term gestation.
- Leaking of amniotic fluid, prolonged or premature rupture of membranes, which are risk factors for neonatal infections.

Dependence on drugs

The mother who has dependence on drugs poses considerable problems during labor, with increased risk to both the mother and the fetus. If the mother begins labor and is currently using illicit drugs, she may be uncooperative, drug seeking, lethargic, or hyperactive, depending on the substance. She may be in danger of developing withdrawal symptoms, which increase risk to the fetus. Drug addicts typically have increased risk of infections, such as hepatitis, HIV/AIDS, and other sexually transmitted diseases. Ideally, the mother's dependence was identified prior to labor and the mother maintained with either methadone or buprenorphine, which can prevent withdrawal and pose a lower risk to the fetus. Both treatments require careful and ongoing monitoring to ensure compliance after a period of stabilization (usually 2 to 3 days). During labor and delivery, those women maintained on methadone or buprenorphine should use those drugs for pain control with careful monitoring to avoid overmedicating.

Induction of labor

Induction of labor stimulates uterine contractions to speed birth and may be done for many conditions, including diabetes mellitus, pre-eclampsia, post-term gestation, mild *abruptio placentae*, oligohydramnios, and poor biophysical profile. Induction is contraindicated with abnormal fetal heart rate patters, breech or uncertain presentation, multiple gestation, maternal heart disease or hypertension, and polyhydramnios. Common induction methods include:

- Stripping/sweeping amniotic membrane: A gloved finger is inserted through the cervical os and rotated (360°) two times to separate the amniotic membrane from the lower part of the uterus in order to release prostaglandins and stimulate contractions. Although not always effective, labor usually begins in 24-48 hours.

- Oxytocin infusion: Oxytocin (Pitocin®) is used to stimulate contractions of the uterus for induction of labor, but risks include over-stimulating the uterus, causing too frequent/intense contractions as well as uterine rupture and water intoxication.

Complementary methods: These methods include sexual intercourse, nipple stimulation, and herbal/homeopathic preparations. These methods have few negative effects.

Caesarean section

Indications

Caesarean sections are done if there is increased risk of uterine rupture, maternal hemorrhage, dystocia including fetal-pelvic disproportion and breech presentation, active herpes infection, and emergent situations, such as fetal distress or impending maternal death. Regional anesthesia (spinal, epidural) is associated with lower mortality than general anesthesia, so it is the preferred anesthetic approach. Additionally, there is less fetal depression, reduced risk of maternal pulmonary aspiration, and an opportunity to provide neuraxial analgesia for postoperative pain relief. Regional anesthesia must provide a T4 sensory level, which causes a high sympathetic blockade. In some cases, general anesthesia may be administered for Caesarean section although the risks to the mother are intensified, so general anesthesia is usually limited to emergent situations in which the mother or fetus are at risk:

- Fetal distress during 2nd stage of labor.
- Tetanic uterine contractions
- Patient confused and uncontrollable and unable to cooperate (such as psychiatric patients).
- Inverted uterus.
- Retained placenta.
- Breech extraction or other position requiring version and extraction.

Cephalopelvic/fetopelvic disproportion

Cephalopelvic/fetopelvic disproportion is usually diagnosed when labor does not progress although in rare cases it may be diagnosed prior to labor. It may relate to pelvic diameters that are too small (most common with android and platypelloid pelvic types) or contractures of the pelvic inlet (<10 cm anteroposterior diameter or <12 cm transverse diameter), contracted midpelvis, or contracted outlet (<8 cm interischial tuberous diameter). Rarely is this disproportion caused by excessive fetal size as most fetuses are within normal size and weight limits. Usually labor is extended, and premature rupture of the membranes occurs, increasing danger of cord prolapse. The fetal head is often markedly molded and continued pressure can cause neurological injury or even death of the fetus if the labor continues and the fetus cannot be delivered. However, when labor fails to progress, the mother is usually given a Caesarean section (≤ 2 hours of labor onset) to prevent further injury to the fetus.

Fetal malpresentation

Cephalic (Variation in normal cephalic/ flexed neck presentation.):

- Military - The head is erect and neck not flexed, but this poses little problem because flexion often occurs as the head descends.
- Brow - The neck is extended so that the brow presents first. This presentation may relate to SGA, LGA, hydramnios, and uterine or fetal anomalies. Brow presentation,

with the largest diameter (about 13.5cm), increases fetal mortality because of birth trauma, which can include compression of the neck and cerebrum and tracheal and laryngeal damage. Vaginal delivery with episiotomy or Caesarean is usually required.
- Face - The neck is severely extended so that the face presents first (about 9.5 cm diameter). This often prolongs labor and may result in increased edema of the fetus and trauma to the neck and internal structures. The neonate usually has bruising in the facial skin.

Breech, shoulder, and compound:
- Breech - This occurs in 4% of births and is frequently related to early labor and delivery (25% at 25-26 weeks gestation). Frank breech (buttocks presentation with legs extended upward) is most common, but single or double footling breech or complete breech (buttocks presentation with legs flexed) can occur. Breech presentation is most common with placenta previa, hydramnios, fetal anomalies, and multiple gestations. Cord prolapse is more likely. Head trauma may occur because molding does not occur, and the head can become entrapped. Mortality and morbidity are reduced with Caesarean section, especially with low or high fetal weight, hyperextension of neck (>90°), fetal anomalies, and pelvic disproportion.
- Shoulder - This transverse lie poses extreme risk of uterine rupture. The fetus cannot be delivered, and Caesarean section is required.
- Compound - Two presenting parts, such as the head and a hand, increasing chances of laceration. With fetal distress or uterine dysfunction, Caesarean section is required.

Delivery

Management of vaginal delivery

Expulsive period

During the expulsive period of delivery, the mother will need to be coached so as to achieve effective pushing effort. Two types of pushing are effective: Open glottis physiologic pushing, and closed glottis (Valsalva) pushing. The mother should be coached on the method most effective for her. During crowning, the mother should be instructed to "pant like a puppy." The integrity of the perineum needs to be taken into consideration. Most mothers would like to avoid an episiotomy if at all possible; however, there are several factors that may require episiotomy:
- Fetal malposition.
- Anticipation of the delivery of a large baby.
- Possibility of shoulder dystocia (where the anterior shoulder cannot pass below the symphysis pubis).
- Poor elasticity of the perineal tissue.
- Difficulty in maintaining adequate control of the patient's expulsive efforts.

Placenta

The placenta will generally deliver 5-30 minutes after delivery of the fetus. The mechanism of placental separation starts with the change in the size of the uterus, then proceeds by the formation of a hematoma between the placenta and uterine wall, the separation of the placenta, the descent of the placenta through the lower uterine segment and vagina, and then expulsion. Signs and symptoms of placental separation include a sudden increase in vaginal bleeding, lengthening of the umbilical cord, and the rising of the uterus in the abdomen. Management of placental delivery includes obtaining cord blood samples after the cord is clamped, inspecting the cord for the number of vessels, and avoiding uterine massage and cord traction until the placenta is separated. Pushing by the mother may assist in expulsion of the placenta. If membranes follow the placenta, one should hold the placenta and roll over and over until the membranes are delivered.

Spinal anesthesia/Saddle block

A saddle block, or spinal anesthesia, is usually given just before vaginal delivery to provide rapid perineal anesthesia. Spinal blocks are avoided during labor because they interfere with motor function. Because of this, other agents may be used during labor. Prior to receiving the spinal anesthesia, the patient is given a bolus of 500-1000 mL fluid. With the patient in sitting position, a very small spinal needle (to prevent CSF leakage and post-spinal headache) is inserted into the subarachnoid space. Local anesthetics used include hyperbaric tetracaine, bupivacaine, or lidocaine, often with the addition of fentanyl or sufentanil to potentiate the effect. The agents are administered between contractions over about 30 seconds. The patient remains sitting for 3 minutes and then is placed in lithotomy position with left uterine displacement to prepare for delivery.

Placental abnormalities/variations

Placental abnormalities/variations are discussed below:

- Battledore - Cord is attached at the periphery of the placenta, usually of no clinical concern. Occurs in up to a third of twin pregnancies.
- Succenturiate lobed - An accessory placenta is within the fetal sac and maintains vascular connections with the main placenta, sometimes resulting in retained placental tissue or hemorrhage, especially if large.
- Velamentous cord insertion - Cord inserts into the membranes rather than the middle of the placenta, traveling through the chorion and amnion to reach the placenta, leaving exposed unprotected vessels. This can cause shearing of the blood vessels during delivery, leading to hemorrhage.
- Circumvallate - A fibrous band of tissue, caused by a double layer of chorion and amnion, appears on the fetal side of the placenta, resulting in deep implantation, but is usual of no clinical concern.

Birthing positions

There are many different birthing positions:

- Hands and knees - Increases perineal relaxation, reducing lacerations and need for episiotomy and facilitating birth with shoulder dystocia; Improves circulation to placenta and umbilical cord; Relieves discomfort of "back labor" but may be fatiguing. Prevents face-to-face contact with mother; Prevents use of instruments, so positional change sometimes required. Prevents mother from viewing birth. Provide pillows for support under chest and upper thighs.
- Left lateral Sims' - Increases perineal relaxation, reducing need for episiotomy. Prevents compromise of peripheral venous return. Slows fetal descent. Prevents mother from viewing birth. Increases comfort. Reduces danger of aspiration.

Requires repositioning if forceps needed or repair of episiotomy. Position mother so that upper leg is supported by pillows, the bed, or partner.

- Semi-Fowler's - Prevents compromise of peripheral venous return. Allows mother to view birth. Decreases perineal relaxation if legs are spread widely. Does not make use of gravity assist, so often used in later stages of labor. Increases mother's comfort level, especially for long labors. Provide adequate support for upper body, legs, and feet using pillows and changing bed position.
- Sitting (birthing bed) - Speeds fetal descent because of pull of gravity. Prevents compromise of peripheral venous return. Allows mother to change leg positions. Allows mother to view birth. Allows a supported sitting position. Provide adequate support for lower extremities.
- Sitting (birthing chair/stool) - Speeds fetal descent and delivery. Reduces need for operative procedures. Prevents compromise of peripheral venous return. Allows mother to view birth. Prevents back support (stool). Reduces pain of "back labor". Allow mother to change position to increase comfort.
- Squatting - Increases pelvic outlet. Speeds fetal descent and delivery. May shorten second stage of labor. Decreases attendant's view of and access to perineum. Increases difficulty of monitoring fetal status and instrument use. Increases perineal edema. Provide birthing bar for mother to hold onto. Provide balance support.
- Recumbent - Allows maintenance of sterile field, good access and view of perineum, and ease of episiotomy. Decreases maternal blood pressure. Increases pressure on diaphragm and maternal dyspnea. Increases risk of laceration and need for episiotomy. Increases risk of aspiration. May interfere with intensity and frequency of uterine contractions. Increases maternal discomfort. Allows mother to view birth. Avoid use of stirrups if possible or ensure they are not causing pressure on lower extremities. Monitor circulation and provide support for legs.

Immediate care of the neonate

Transition and first period of reactivity

This neonate's transition period begins immediately after the delivery when the infant stabilizes and adjusts to life outside of the womb. This involves three stages: the first period of reactivity, the period of unresponsive sleep and the second period of reactivity; however, these stages may undergo alteration if there is significant stress during labor and/or delivery. To minimize stress to the infant, contact with the mother should be maintained, and examinations and/or procedures should be delayed if appropriate.

- First period of reactivity - This period begins immediately after delivery and lasts about 30 minutes. Assessment should show heartbeat and respirations near the upper limits of normal, respiratory rales for about 20 minutes, alertness, the startle reflex and crying. Breastfeeding should be encouraged during this period as it helps the blood glucose level to drop to normal within 90 minutes after delivery.
- Period of unresponsive sleep - This period occurs after the first period of reactivity and lasts from 30 minutes after birth to 2 hours after birth. During this period, the heart rate decreases to less than 140 bpm, a heart murmur may be present due to incomplete closure of the ductus arteriosus and the respirations slow and become more regular.

- Second period of reactivity - This period lasts from two to six hours after birth. During this time, the heart rate may become unstable and changing, there may be rapid changes in skin color, and the respirations slow to less than 60 per minute; however, the rales should clear by this time. The infant may be interested in feeding, which will help prevent hypoglycemia, stimulate a bowel movement, and prevent jaundice.

Rapid assessment

The infant should be given a rapid assessment within seconds of birth to determine if the infant is at term, if the amniotic fluid is clear, if there is muscle tone, and if there are respirations or crying. If any of these conditions are not met, then the child should be placed under radiant heat and further resuscitation done. The basic steps to resuscitation include:

- Warming the infant after drying.
- Positioning the infant and clearing the airway if necessary.
- Stimulating and repositioning the infant.

The child should be evaluated throughout the initial procedures:

- Respirations: Rate and character of respirations should be noted as well as observation of chest wall movement.
- Heart rate: Should be >100 bpm, assessed with stethoscope or at the base of the umbilical cord.

Times and types of assessment

The neonate should undergo three different types of physical assessment:

- Immediate: The first examination is done in the delivery room to determine the need for resuscitation or other intervention. This includes Apgar assessment.
- 1-4 hours after birth: The second examination includes gestational age assessment, which must be completed within 24 hours for accuracy, and brief physical assessment to determine if there are any problems that might place the infant at risk. This includes assessment of respiratory and cardiac status, cord color, skin color, and movement. The Modified Ballard scoring system is often used.
- ≥24 hours after birth (or prior to discharge): The final examination should include a complete physical and behavioral assessment that includes all systems and evaluation of reflexes. All weights and measurements are taken and reviewed. This exam requires observation, palpation, and auscultation. In some cases, instead of a separate examination at 1-4 hours, only this complete physical examination is completed.

Providing warmth

Infants have poor temperature regulation ability, particularly preterm infants who lack brown fat, which is one of the body's tools to regulate body temperature, so providing warmth is critical as a component of resuscitation. An infant who is just seconds old and wet will need aggressive measures to keep it warm while any resuscitation efforts are being initiated. Infants lose heat through their head so one of the first steps should be to place a hat on the head. The infant should be placed under a radiant heater and vigorous drying with warmed blankets should begin. Often this stimulation, drying and warming is all that is needed to establish a regular respiration pattern in the neonate. Preterm infants weighing <1500 grams should be placed in a plastic bag (made specifically for this purpose) up to the height of the shoulders to prevent cold shock. A term infant with no apparent distress can be placed on the mother's chest and covered with a warm blanket.

APGAR delivery room assessment

Dr. Virginia Apgar developed the APGAR test in 1952. APGAR stands for **A**ppearance, **P**ulse, **G**rimace, **A**ctivity, and **R**espiration. The APGAR is the first test given to a newborn. It is used as a quick evaluation of a newborn's physical condition to determine if any emergency medical care is needed and is administered 1 minute and 5 minutes after birth. The test is administered more than once, as the baby's condition may change rapidly. It may be administered for a third time 10 minutes after birth if needed. The baby is rated on the five subscales and scores added together. A total score of ≥7 is a sign of good health:

- Appearance (Skin Color):
    - Cyanotic or pallor over entire body – 0
    - Normal, except for the extremities – 1
    - Entire body normal – 2
- Pulse (Heart Rate):
    - Absent - 0
    - <100 bpm - 1
    - >100 bpm – 2
- Grimace (Reflex Irritability):
    - Unresponsive - 0
    - Grimace – 1
    - Infant sneezes, coughs, and recoils – 2
- Activity (Muscle Tone):
    - Absent - 0
    - Flexed limbs – 1
    - Infant moves freely – 2
- Respiration (Breathing Rate and Effort):
    - Absent – 0
    - Bradypnea, dyspnea – 1
    - Good breathing and crying - 2

Establishing airway

To establish an airway, the infant is placed supine with the head slightly extended in the "sniffing" position. A small neck roll may be placed under the shoulders to maintain this position in a very small premature infant. Once the proper position is established, the mouth and nose is suctioned (mouth first to prevent reflex inspiration of secretions when nose suctioned) with a bulb syringe or catheter if necessary. The infant's head can be turned momentarily to the side to allow secretions to pool in the cheek where they can be more easily suctioned and removed to establish the airway. Stimulating the newborn is often all that is needed to initiate spontaneous respirations in the neonate. This tactile stimulation can be accomplished by gently rubbing the back or trunk of the infant. Another technique used to provide stimulation is flicking or rubbing the soles of the feet. Slapping neonates as stimulation is no longer practiced and should NOT be used.

ABCs of infant resuscitation

The ABC's of resuscitation are a device to help remember what order to do which steps of the resuscitation process. In this device, the letters stand for as follows:

- A—Airway - An airway should be established as the very first thing tended to, if there is no airway, air cannot be moved during resuscitation attempts. This step includes clearing the mouth and nose of secretions, and properly positioning the infant in the "sniff" position.
- B—Breathing - This step involves initiating breathing after the airway has been established; this can be done with stimulation, supplemental oxygen or through artificial ventilation.
- C—Circulation - Once an airway and breathing have been established, then the circulation is considered; chest compressions may be indicated here or the administration of volume expanders and possibly epinephrine.

Meconium in amniotic fluid

When meconium is present in the amniotic fluid, the following steps should be taken immediately following birth to avoid meconium aspiration syndrome:

- If the infant is crying and showing no signs of distress, the mouth, nose and throat should be suctioned with a suction catheter and the usual steps of drying and stimulation completed.
- If the infant shows signs of respiratory distress in the presence of meconium stained fluid, the infant should be immediately intubated with an endotracheal tube for the purpose of suctioning the trachea. Once intubated, the trachea can be suctioned with a large catheter attached to wall suction.
- Once the airway has been adequately suctioned and cleared, the stomach may need to be suctioned as well in order to prevent the regurgitation of the swallowed meconium. Meconium that is swallowed and then regurgitated can be aspirated into the lungs.

Facilitating the attachment progress

Facilitating the attachment process begins before delivery by educating the mother about bonding and the importance of early and close contact with her infant. Ensuring skin-to-skin contact within the first hour is especially important, but different approaches are used:

- If the neonate appears stable at delivery, he/she should be placed on the mother's abdomen for drying and initial assessment and then placed between the mother's breasts and covered with a blanket to prevent temperature loss. Weighing, measuring, and bathing the infant is deferred.
- The neonate may be assessed in a warmer, dried, diapered, weighed and measured and then placed between the mother's breasts.
- After delivery, the neonate should be held with skin-to-skin contact as soon as possible and as often as possible.
- If the mother is breastfeeding, the neonate should start nursing within 30 to 60 minutes of delivery.

Caesarean birth

Anesthesia
Caesarean births have a higher mortality rate than vaginal births, with complications including infection, blood clots, and hemorrhage. The Caesarean is usually done with a regional (spinal, epidural) anesthetic rather than general anesthetic because general anesthesia poses more risks to the mother and causes more fetal depression. Regional anesthesia must provide a T4 sensory level (high sympathetic blockade). An opioid and nitrous oxide or propofol may be administered after the delivery is complete to provide amnesia and prevent recall. If the mother was non-fasting or aspiration is a concern, an orogastric tube may be inserted and aspiration of stomach contents done to reduce the chance of aspiration during emergence from general anesthesia. Additionally, the patient should be extubated only after awake. Blood loss with Caesarean section is about 1000 mL, so fluid replacement must balance estimated loss.

Skin and uterine incisions
Caesarean births require two different types of incisions. Skin incisions may be transverse or vertical. Transverse incisions leave less obvious scarring but delivery takes longer. Likewise, uterine incisions may be vertical or transverse, but not always the same as the skin incision:

- Kerr incision: The most common uterine incision is the transverse lower uterine incision because the uterus is thinnest, bleeding is less, repair is easier, adhesion development is less, bladder dissection is less, and risk of rupture with subsequent pregnancies decreases; however, the size is restricted by major vessels on the sides, and the incision requires more time.
- Sellheim incision: Vertical incision in the lower uterus is usually used for multiple gestation, malpresentations, placenta previa, macrosomia, and preterm deliveries because it allows better access and faster delivery, but this approach carries a greater risk of rupture with subsequent pregnancies (which then require C-section), and requires more dissection of the bladder.

First Postpartal Hour

Immediate care of the mother

C-section
The initial assessments of the mother who has had a Caesarean section and the neonate are similar to vaginal birth, but the mother also must recover from a surgical procedure and anesthesia. Immediate postoperative care during the first postpartal hour includes the following:

- VS are checked every 5 minutes until stable and then every 15 minutes for one hour; finally, VS are checked every 30 minutes until the mother is released from the recovery area.
- The abdominal dressing and perineal pad should be checked every 15 minutes for bleeding for the first hour and the fundus gently palpated with a hand supporting the incisional area.
- IV oxytocin is administered to promote contraction of the uterine muscles.

- General anesthesia: The patient is positioned on her side and turned every 2 hours for 24 hours.
- Epidural or spinal anesthesia: The level of anesthesia checked every 15 minutes.
- Intake and output are monitored and urine is checked for signs of blood (indicating bladder trauma).
- Analgesia is given as indicated to control pain.

Immediate care of the mother after vaginal delivery

Maternal monitoring during the first postpartal hour consists of the following:

- Vital signs:
  - VS should be checked every 15 minutes and evaluated in relation to baseline VS and VS prior to delivery.
  - Normal BP varies between 90-140/60-90.
  - Falling BP and increased pulse may indicate uterine bleeding.
  - Pulse (60-90) is usually slightly decreased from that found during labor.
  - Respirations should be relaxed and not labored usually ranging 12-20/min.
- Temperature: Slight temperature elevation is normal immediately after delivery (≤100.4) but this should return to normal by 24 hour.
- Alertness: The mother should be awake, alert, responsive, and able to hold infant.
- Fundus:
  - The fundus is palpated to determine if it is firm, midline, and in the expected position (umbilicus).
  - A boggy fundus may indicate uterine bleeding.
  - Bladder distention may cause the fundus to deviate from midline.
- Lochia:
  - The lochia should be checked every 15 minutes for signs of excess bleeding, such as copious discharge or large clots.
  - The lochia must be observed while the fundus is massaged to determine if there is free flow of blood or expulsion of clots, which may indicate hemorrhage.
  - The lochia rubra should be present with a moderate amount of discharge, <1 perineal pad/hr.
- Perineum:
  - The perineal area should be examined and amount of swelling and bruising noted as well as condition of episiotomy (if present) and sutures.
  - Severe perineal/rectal pain requires further examination.
- Bladder:
  - The bladder should be palpated to determine if it is distended.
  - The mother should be given the opportunity to urinate within the first hour after delivery before catheterization is considered.
  - Mother should spontaneously urinate >100 mL clear urine with no distention noted after urination.
- Rectum:
  - The rectum should be examined for the presence of tearing or hemorrhoids.
  - No severe rectal pain should be present.
  - If hemorrhoids are present, engorgement must be reported to physician, especially if ≥2 cm in size.

- Pain:
  - The mother should have only mild pain, <3 on 1-10 scale.
  - Severe pain requires further examination to determine cause.
  - Analgesia should be provided to control pain.
- Legs/feet:
  - The feet and legs should be warm and pulses palpable.
  - Edema, which may have been present before delivery, should remain stable or decrease.
- Anesthesia: If the mother had an anesthetic, such as epidural or spinal, the level of anesthesia should be assessed every 15 minutes.

Uterine involution

The normal uterus weighs about 70-100 g with a capacity of 5 mL. During pregnancy, the uterus increases in weight to 1000 g with capacity of 5000 mL. After delivery, the uterus weight decreases to 500 g by the end of the first week, 300 by the second, and 100 by the third. Uterine involution (the process of the uterus returning to the pre-pregnant state) begins immediately after the placenta separates. A number of changes occur over the first 3 weeks (except for the placental site, which takes 6 to 7 weeks to heal over):

- Estrogen and progesterone levels drop markedly, causing cells to atrophy and reversing hyperplasia.
- Autolysis occurs as proteolytic enzymes are released and macrophages migrate to the uterus.
- The spongy layer of decidua sloughs off as lochia.
- The basal layer of decidua separates into two layers within 48-72 hours with the outer layer becoming necrotic and sloughing off as lochia and the inner layer providing the base for the new endometrium.

Intrapartal Period (Normal Labor)

Stages of labor and delivery

The stages of labor present somewhat differently from one woman to another and in multipara and nullipara.

First stage

This stage signals onset of labor with regular contractions and proceeds until the cervix is fully dilated. There are 3 phases:

- Latent: This early phase may persist for 8.5 hours for nullipara and 5.3 hours for the multipara. The cervix begins to dilate (≤3 cm) and contractions may occur every 3-30 minutes, lasting 20-40 seconds. The intensity of the contractions is usually mild to moderate (25-40 mm Hg per intrauterine pressure catheter—IUPC). The mother is usually able to cope with discomfort and may feel some anxiety.
- Active: This phase may persist for 4.5 hrs in the nullipara but 2.5 hours in the multipara. The cervix dilates to 4-7 cm (1.2 cm/hr for nullipara and 1.5 cm/hr for multipara) with contractions increasing in frequency every 1-5 minutes with duration 40-60 seconds. The intensity is moderate to strong (50-70 mm Hg per IUPC) and anxiety and pain increase.
- Transition: This phase may persist for 3.6 hours for the nullipara and ≤1 hour for the multipara although this duration may increase an hour with epidural anesthesia. The cervix becomes fully dilated to 8-10 cm with frequent contractions every 1.5-2 minutes lasting 60-90 seconds. The intensity is strong by palpation and 70-90 mm Hg per IUPC. During this stage, the mother may experience much anxiety and pain and the feeling that bearing down or contractions will tear her apart. Cervical dilation slows between 8-10 cm and fetal descent increases (1 cm/hr for nullipara and 2 cm/hr for multipara). Mothers frequently request pain medication and may hyperventilate, have difficulty following directions, cry or moan, become very restless, hiccup, belch or vomit, and complain of rectal pressure.

Second stage

The second stage of labor begins when the cervix is fully dilated and ends with delivery. This stage usually lasts for about 2 hours for the nullipara but only 15 minutes for the multipara. Frequent contractions continue every 1.5-2 minutes and last 60-90 seconds (as in transition phases of stage 1), and intensity if very strong by palpation and 70-100 mm Hg by UIPC. As the fetal head descends, it applies pressure to the sacral and obturator nerves, causing an intense urge to bear down. The perineum begins to bulge and flatten out and bloody show increases. The mother often feels severe pain and burning in the perineal area. The fetal head crowns as delivery is imminent. The perineum thins as the fetal head distends the vulva and the anus, sometimes causing stool to be expelled. The head is born and then the shoulders and body in a spontaneous (non-breech) birth.

Third and fourth stages

The third stage of labor commences after the delivery of the infant and ends after the placenta is delivered. After delivery, strong uterine contractions decrease surface area of placental attachment, causing separation, which is accompanied by bleeding and formation of a hematoma between the decidua and the placental tissue. Finally, the placental membrane peels off of the uterine wall. Signs of placental separation usually occur between 5 and 30 minutes after birth:

- Globular-shaped uterus.
- Fundus rises in the abdomen.
- Increased gush or trickling of blood.
- Umbilical cord protrudes further from the vagina.

A placenta is considered retained if it has not separated in over 30 minutes after delivery. The fourth stage is the time period extending from 1-4 hours after birth during which the mother's body goes through physiologic readjustment. Blood is redistributed and this, coupled with 250-400 mL blood loss, contributes to moderate hypotension and tachycardia. The uterus stays contracted, and the fundus is usually midline between the symphysis pubis and umbilicus.

Assessing the progress of labor and vital signs

Assessments during the first stage of labor consist of the following:

- Initial admission exam:
    - Contractions: Frequency and duration and changes are noted since onset.
    - Cervical exam: Dilatation may vary from 1 to 10 cm with nullipara dilatation averaging 1.2 cm/hr and multipara averaging 1.5 cm/hr. Effacement varies from 0 to 100%. Fetal descent may range from +4 to -4.
- Latent phase:
    - Check baseline VS and then monitor every hour if they are stable (90-140/60-90) or every 15 minutes if unstable or elevating >30 mm Hg systolic/>15 mm Hg diastolic over baseline.
    - Monitor temperature every 4 hours. If it is >37.6 °C or if membranes rupture, monitor every 2 hours.
    - Monitor uterine contractions every 30 minutes (usually occur every 5 to 10 minutes with a duration of 15 to 40 seconds, mild intensity.).
    - Monitor FHR every 60 minutes for low risk mothers and every 30 minutes for high risk if FHR remains within normal range (110-160). If FHR is unstable, use continuous monitoring.
- Active phase:
    - Check VS every hour if they are stable or every 15 minutes if unstable.
    - Monitor temperature every 4 hours. If it is >37.6 °C or if membranes rupture, monitor every 2 hours.
    - Monitor uterine contractions every 15 to 30 minutes (usually occur every 2 to 3 minutes with a duration of 60 seconds, moderate intensity).
    - Monitor FHR every 30 minutes for low risk mothers and every 15 minutes for high risk mothers if FHR is within normal range. Institute interventions as necessary if FHR is unstable.
    - Monitor mother's comfort level and coping mechanisms.
    - Monitor response to analgesia/anesthesia.
- Transition phase:
    - Check VS every 30 minutes.

- Monitor uterine contractions every 15 minutes (usually occur every 2 minutes with a duration of 60 to 75 seconds, strong intensity).
- Monitor bladder distention. Use a straight cath if the mother is unable to urinate.
- Continue monitoring comfort level, coping mechanisms, and response to analgesia/anesthesia.

Assessments during the second and third stages of labor consist of the following:

- Second stage:
    - Check VS every 5 to 15 minutes.
    - Monitor uterine contractions continuously
    - Monitor FHR every 15 minutes for low risk mothers and every 5 minutes for high risk mothers. If unstable, monitor VS continuously.
    - Monitor fetal descent.
    - Monitor mother's comfort level and coping mechanisms.
    - Monitor response to analgesia, anesthesia.
    - Monitor bladder distention. Use a straight cath if the mother is unable to urinate.
- Third stage
    - Check VS every 5 minutes.
    - Continue to monitor all aspects of labor and delivery.
    - Monitor uterine contractions every few minutes or as indicated until the placenta is delivered.
    - Monitor response to analgesia, anesthesia (epidural, spinal).
    - Provide support during pudendal local anesthesia and episiotomy if indicated.
    - Monitor bladder distention. Use a straight cath if the mother is unable to urinate.

Support available during labor

<u>Birth plan</u>
Having a birth plan prepared can alleviate much of the stress associated with labor because it allows the mother and her partner to make decisions in advance about what she wants during labor and delivery. The following elements can be planned by the mother in advance:

- Labor:
    - Specific preferences regarding ambulation during the labor procedure and IVs or oral fluids
    - May also indicate how frequently the mother wants vaginal exams.
- Fetal monitoring: Desire for continuous fetal monitoring or intermittent
- Induction: Condition under which induction procedures or other procedures to speed up labor, such as artificial rupturing of the membranes, are acceptable.
- Anesthesia/comfort measures:
    - Preferences for natural childbirth, opiates only, epidural, or spinal anesthesia.
    - May include any birth preparation methods the mother plans to use, such as Lamaze.
- Surgical interventions: Specific conditions for C-section or episiotomy.

- Delivery: Instructions regarding positioning, pushing, mirror, support (partner, friend, husband), and immediate care of newborn.
- Postpartal period: Includes preferences regarding cutting cord, rooming in, nursery care, private or shared room, breastfeeding, supplementary feeding, and disposing/donating cord blood.

Progressive relaxation and vocalization

Progressive relaxation is one method to help the mother relax her muscles and relieve tension so that uterine contractions are more effective. Progressive relaxation involves first tightening muscles and holding the tension for a few seconds and then relaxing them, concentrating on the difference in feeling between the tense and relaxed muscle states and imagining the tension flowing out of the muscles. Relaxation is usually done bilaterally, starting with the feet and moving upward through the muscles of the lower legs, the hands, the lower arms, the upper arms, and finally the abdomen and chest, the neck, and the face. Vocalization is a technique that encourages the woman to make sounds during contractions in order to relieve tension and relax muscles. The woman is coached to drop her jaw and try to make low-pitched (masculine sounding) moans as this method opens the glottis and makes breathing easier. High-pitched moaning should be avoided as it may increase tension.

Touch relaxation

Touch relaxation requires a coach and is generally practiced prior to onset of labor. The mother learns to relax her muscles in response to touch—first her partner's and later doctors' and nurses'. In this technique, the mother tightens a small area of muscles, and her coach gently strokes the area, "pulling" the tension away as the mother immediately relaxes the muscles at the first touch. Strokes are generally in a downward direction. Touch relaxation follows a specific sequence, and a printed guide may be helpful for the woman and her coach. The sequence of contracting and relaxing begins with the scalp and eyebrows, the rest of the face and jaw, the shoulder blades, abdomen, thighs, legs, and arms. After the initial sequence, the mother lies on her side, tightening the back of the neck, which the coach then strokes and massages. Then, she curls into fetal position and tightens the upper back, lower back, and buttocks.

Dissociation relaxation

Dissociation relaxation is a method that teaches the mother to tighten just one set of voluntary muscles and relax the rest (neuromuscular dissociation) to prepare the mother to relax all voluntary muscles during uterine contractions. This technique uses discomfort to help the mother dissociate from the pain. For example, the partner may grasp the upper arms and rotate the skin outward to create a burning sensation in the muscles or pinch an area of the inner thigh (being careful not to injure the woman or cause real pain). Then, the woman relaxes other muscles in a sequence of contracting, holding, and relaxing. The partner touches the relaxed muscles to check relaxation. The usual sequence is right arm, left arm, right leg, left leg, both arms, both legs, right arm and leg, and finally left arm and leg.

Visualization

There are a number of methods used for visualization. Some include audiotapes with guided imagery, such as self-hypnosis tapes, but the pregnant woman can be taught basic techniques that include:

- Lie on back or left side (preferred) in a quiet place (if possible), eliminating unnecessary distractions
- Concentrate on breathing while taking long slow breaths.
- Close the eyes to shut out distractions and create an image in the mind of the place or situation desired.
- Concentrate on that image, engaging as many senses as possible and imaging details.
- If the mind wanders, breathe deeply and bring consciousness back to the image or concentrate on breathing for a few moments and then return to the imagery.
- End with positive imagery.

Sometimes, women in labor are resistive at first or have a hard time maintaining focus, so guiding them through visualization for the first few times can be helpful.

Positioning, hydrotherapy, and comfort

Mothers are often encouraged to ambulate during the first stage of labor, but if the FHR is not reassuring or if the membranes are ruptured, the mother may be confined to bed or chair. In that case, she should be helped to turn at least every hour or to sit in a warm shower or rocking chair to increase relaxation and relieve discomfort. If in bed, the body, arms, and legs should be supported comfortably with pillows or bolsters with joints slightly flexed. If the mother prefers the supine position, the head of the bed should be elevated to at least 30° and support placed under the lower back to relieve uterine pressure on the vena cava. Shower, warm bath, and whirlpool all help to relax the mother and reduce discomfort. Tub bath and whirlpool, however, should be avoided if the membranes have ruptured. Increased vaginal discharge can cause odor and discomfort, so the perineal pad should be changed at least every hour and the perineum gently washed with warm water and soap to remove secretions. Diaphoresis, the effort expended during labor, and breathing patterns often cause the mother to feel thirsty and complain of dry mouth. If allowed, clear fluids should be offered; otherwise, ice chips or hard candy may be used.

Increased perspiration and amniotic leakage often leave the woman's bedclothes damp and cold, so frequent gown and linen changes should be done. Underpads can be placed under the buttocks and changed frequently as they are more easily changed than the bottom sheet. A cool damp cloth on the forehead may be soothing. The mother may be unable to completely empty the bladder because of fetal pressure or discomfort, but a distended bladder will add to her discomfort during contractions. The mother should be encouraged to try urinating every 1 to 2 hours preferably on the toilet as it may be more difficult to empty the bladder on a bedpan. If the mother is unable to urinate or completely empty her bladder and her bladder remains distended, a straight catheterization may be necessary, although repeated catheterizations increase the risk of infection. Sitting with the legs spread apart on a birthing ball and slowly rocking back and forth helps to increase pelvic diameter and facilitate fetal descent. The mother should not be left unattended while on the ball as she may lose balance or fall.

Opioids and sedatives

Opioids and sedatives are usually given only in the early stages of labor, sometimes with PAC, because they readily cross the placental barrier and can cause central nervous system depression in the fetus. This depression can persist after delivery, especially in premature infants, affecting Apgar scores. Some drugs, such as morphine and benzodiazepines, are avoided because of excessive fetal depression. Drugs used include:

- Meperidine (1-25 mg IV or 25-50 IM to maximum 100 mg) is the most common. IV onset is 1-20 minutes and IM 1-3 hour, and its use is limited to >4 hours before delivery.
- Fentanyl (25-100 μg/hr IV) has shorter onset (3-10 minutes) with one-hour duration and causes less fetal depression.
- Butorphanol 1-2 mg or nalbuphine 10-20 mg IV or IM cause little respiratory effect and provide adequate relief of pain but may result in excessive sedation if given repeatedly.
- Promethazine (25-50 mg IM) and hydroxyzine may be used in combination with meperidine or alone to provide relief of anxiety and reduce dose of opioid.

Pudendal nerve block

Visceral pain occurs in the first stage of labor from contractions and cervical dilation with afferent impulses entering the spinal cord at T10-T11. However, during the second stage of labor, the stretching of the vagina and perineum caused by descent of the fetus causes somatic pain with impulses carried by the pudendal nerves to the spinal cord at S2-S4. Pudendal nerve block is used during the second stage (sometimes along with perineal infiltration) to reduce somatic pain when neuraxial blocks are contraindicated and for episiotomy and relaxation of the pelvic floor for forceps delivery. With the patient in lithotomy position, a transvaginal or transperineal approach is used to block the nerve. For the transvaginal approach (the most common), a Kobak needle or special guide (Iowa trumpet) is used to prevent inadvertent injection into the fetal head. Anesthetic agents include 10 mL of 1% lidocaine or 2% chloroprocaine. The transperineal approach may be used if the head is engaged.

Lumbar epidural

The most common form of regional anesthesia/analgesia for labor and delivery is the lumbar epidural. Dilute mixtures of local anesthetic and opioids are combined. The catheter is usually placed early so that it is available when pain relief is needed. At one time, epidurals were delayed until labor was well established, but current trends are to administer earlier if the fetus is in no distress, contractions are 3-4 minutes and persisting at least 60 seconds, and the fetal head is engaged with 3-4 cm of cervical dilation. The catheter is usually placed with the mother in sitting position to ensure sacral spread. Placement is usually at L3-L4 or L4-L5. If inadvertent spinal placement occurs, spinal anesthesia/analgesia may be given or the catheter removed and replaced at a higher level. Most commonly, bupivacaine or ropivacaine (0.0625-0.125%) is given in combination with fentanyl (2-3 μg/ mL) or sufentanil (0.3-0.5 μg/mL). If dilute anesthetic agents are used, the mother may be able to ambulate while receiving the epidural.

Epidural analgesia with opioids

Epidural analgesia with just opioids is also sometimes used during the first stage of labor. Commonly used agents include morphine (5 mg), meperidine (50-100 mg), fentanyl (50-150 μg), and sufentanil (10-20 μg). The duration of analgesia is longer with administration of epidural opioids than with intrathecal, but many of the same problems occur. Low doses of morphine may not provide adequate pain relief and higher doses may cause respiratory depression. Morphine has a slow onset (0.5-1 hour) but provides analgesia for 12-24 hours. Meperidine provides good relief but is short-acting (1-3 hours). Fentanyl and sufentanil both have rapid onset but are also short acting (1-2 hours). Commonly, morphine is combined with fentanyl or sufentanil for fast onset with long duration. The fetus must be monitored carefully if repeated epidural doses of opioids are administered as they can cause fetal depression.

Intrathecal analgesia with opioids

Intrathecal (spinal) analgesia (into the subarachnoid space) with just opioids is sometimes used during the first stage of labor. Commonly used agents include morphine (0.25-0.5 mg), meperidine (10-15 mg), fentanyl, 12.5-15 μg, and sufentanil 92-10 μg). Meperidine is the only agent that has local anesthetic characteristics. Higher doses are needed if spinal opioids are used alone, administered as a single dose or intermittently per catheter, and this can result in higher risk of complications, maternal respiratory depression, and fetal depression. However, if given alone, opioids (except for meperidine) do not provide motor blockade or maternal hypotension, so the mother is able to push. However, the analgesic effect may not be adequate, and side effects (pruritus, nausea, and vomiting) related to the agent may occur. Morphine alone has a slow onset (45-60 minutes) although it provides 4-6 hours of analgesia with spinal administration, but low doses may not provide adequate relief and high doses increase side effects. Morphine is frequently combined with fentanyl for more rapid onset. Commonly, opioids are combined with local anesthetics.

Fetal monitoring

Continuous fetal heart rate monitoring

Fetal heart rate (FHR) monitoring is usually done by electronic fetal monitoring (EFM) as it provides a continuous tracing. FHR can be assessed by auscultation or ultrasound with an abdominal transducer, but tracings can be poor with an active fetus, with maternal movement, and with hydramnios. Intermittent monitoring is usually every 15 minutes in the first stage of labor and every 5 minutes in the second. Internal monitoring requires cervical dilation of ≥2cm so that an electrode can be applied to the fetal presenting part (head or buttocks). Internal scalp electrodes should not be used if the mother has a communicable disease, such as HIV, or with preterm infants. Telemetry with ultrasound or fetal ECG transducers and external uterine pressure transducers can also be used to monitor FHR. This type of battery-operated monitoring can be used while the mother ambulates, as it is less invasive. FHR patterns are evaluated based on a baseline rate (rate for 10 minutes between contractions), usually 110-160 bpm. Bradycardia is a rate <120 bmp; and tachycardia, >160 bpm.

Fetal scalp sampling and stimulation

Fetal scalp sampling involves making a small cut in the fetal scalp and collecting a blood sample. Fetal scalp sampling is used to determine if the fetus is receiving enough oxygen during labor, to measure fetal platelets, and to rule out acidosis. This technique has several limiting factors, such as inadequate cervical dilation, fetal head too high, membranes still intact, or sampling errors due to hematoma of the fetus' scalp. The results of the sampling are normal if greater than 7.25, pre-pathological if between 7.20-to-7.25 and pathological if less than 7.20. The test must be repeated every 20-to-30 minutes because the results are time-limited. Fetal scalp stimulation is done during the vaginal examination by gently massaging the scalp for 15 seconds. The results of scalp stimulation should be an increase in the fetal heart rate of 10 to 15 beats over baseline for 10 to 15 seconds. Failure of the heartbeat to accelerate is an indication of acidosis.

Premature labor

Preterm or premature labor occurs within weeks 20-37. Premature rupture of membrane (PROM) occurs when the membranes rupture before the onset of labor and may lead to premature labor. There are numerous causes for PROM, including infections and digital pelvic exams. When a woman presents in labor, the estimated date of delivery should be obtained by questioning the date of the last menstrual period (LMP) and using a gestation calculator wheel or estimating with Naegele's rule:

- First day LMP minus 3 months plus 7 days = estimated date of delivery.

Fetal viability is very low before 23 weeks of gestation but by 25 weeks, delaying delivery for 2 days can increase survival rates by 10%. Tocolytic drugs, which have many negative side effects, may be used to delay delivery in order to administer glucocorticoids, such as betamethasone or dexamethasone, to improve fetal lung maturity between weeks 24-36.

Tocolysis

Tocolysis suppresses preterm labor and premature birth, sometimes allowing time to administer betamethasone to accelerate maturity of fetal lungs. Tocolytics (some off-label) include:

- Nifedipine a calcium channel blocker that reduces muscle contractility, is most commonly used, as it is more effective and safer than many other drugs. It may increase fetal heart rate (FHR).
- Terbutaline is a β-adrenergic asthma drug that also relaxes the uterine muscle. It may increase FHR.
- Magnesium sulfate is similar in action to terbutaline, but it requires close monitoring for maternal adverse effects. It crosses the placenta, and the neonate may suffer respiratory and motor depression.
- Indomethacin, NSAID that inhibits prostaglandin production can be used up to 32 weeks gestation. It crosses the placenta and can cause reduction in amniotic fluid, leading to fetal distress, especially >32 weeks. Indomethacin can also cause premature closure of the ductus arteriosus.
- Ritodrine is a β-2 agonist that relaxes smooth muscles and can delay delivery for 24-48 hours but may increase fetal heart rate.

Postpartal Period

Maternal Physical Needs

The fundus

The uterus contracts after the placenta is expelled to about grapefruit size with the fundus about midway to two-thirds the distance between the symphysis pubis and the umbilicus. The contraction of the uterus brings the uterine walls together and compresses the vessels to prevent bleeding:

- Over the 6-12 hours after delivery, blood and clots pool in the uterus and the fundus rises midline to the level of the umbilicus where it stays for about 12 hours. A fundus above the umbilicus and boggy indicates excessive bleeding. A high fundus that deviates from midline often indicates a distended bladder.
- By first postpartum day, the fundus is about 1 cm (one finger-width) below the umbilicus.
- The fundus continues to descend about 1 cm per day until it is no longer palpable (usually within 2 weeks).

If a boggy uterus is felt on fundal examination, it should be massaged until the uterus contracts, expels clots and debris, and firms. If it fails to firm, the physician should be notified.

Lochia

Lochia, vaginal discharge after delivery, rids the uterus of remaining debris. The total volume of discharge is about 240 to 480 mL, with discharge decreasing over time. Discharge is usually increased in the morning because of pooling. The lochia should be examined to assess both hemorrhage and uterine involution. The stages are as follows:

- Rubra – (Days 1 to 3 or 4) The lochia is a dark red discharge containing epithelial cells, red and white blood cells, bacteria, decidua shreds, lanugo, vernix caseosa, and sometimes meconium. Clots should not exceed nickel size, as large clots may indicate hemorrhage—although this should be differentiated from bleeding from vaginal lacerations.
- Serosa – (Days 4 to 10) The lochia is a pinkish to brownish discharge containing serous exudate, decidua shreds, red and white blood cells, cervical mucus, and various microorganisms. It gradually lightens as the number of red blood cells decreases.
- Alba – (Persists additional 2-85 days, average 24.) The lochia is a yellowish discharge that contains primarily white blood cells, epithelial cells, decidual cells, fat, mucus, and bacteria. The cervix is closed when lochia alba flow stops, so the danger of infection ceases.

Assessment of breasts

Hormonal changes with birth stimulate the breasts to increase milk production. The mother may feel some increased fullness. The breasts should feel full but not hard on gentle palpation and may be slightly tender. The mother should be advised to avoid sleeping in the prone position as this compresses the breasts and increases the risk of complications, such as a clogged milk duct. Breastfeeding should begin immediately or within 30-60 minutes of birth. Colostrum does not pose a danger to the neonate, even if aspirated, and nursing promotes bonding with the infant and contraction of the uterus. Colostrum, produced the first 2-4 days, is thick and yellow and produced only in teaspoonfuls, but this is adequate for the neonate whose stomach capacity the first day is only 5 to 7 mL. Colostrum provides both antibodies and protein. By day 3, transitional milk is thinning and the stomach capacity is 1 ounce. By day 7, when mature milk is starting to come in, the neonate's stomach capacity is 1.5 to 2 ounces.

Comfort measures

The mother undergoes multiple physiological changes during the puerperium (postpartal period), beginning immediately after birth, but many of the changes may be alleviated by simple comfort measures:

- Hunger - Mothers often feel very hungry after giving birth and may enjoy a light meal. If the mother had a C-section, she may be limited to clear liquids initially but should be progressed to a regular diet as soon as possible.
- Thirst - Because fluids are lost during delivery, the mother often experiences marked thirst, alleviated by providing ample oral fluids to replace those lost. If the mother had a C-section and is receiving IVs, then the rate of replacement must be adequate.
- Chill - Postpartal chill immediately after delivery is common and may relate to neurological or vasomotor changes. The mother should be covered with a warmed blanket and offered warm liquids.
- Diaphoresis - Perspiration increases during the puerperium to help eliminate excess fluid and waste products, but the mother may wake up drenched in sweat at night. The mother should be provided dry gown and linens and protected from chilling.
- Afterpains - With a first pregnancy, the uterus usually remains contracted after delivery, but with subsequent pregnancies or complications, such as hydramnios or retention of clots or placental tissue, the uterus may alternate between contraction and relaxation, causing severe cramp-like afterpains in the 2-3 days after delivery. Additionally, if the mother receives oxytocin to stimulate contractions, this may increase discomfort. Breastfeeding naturally stimulates release of oxytocin, so nursing may cause afterpains. Analgesic agents such as acetaminophen or ibuprofen, especially an hour before nursing and at bedtime, may relieve discomfort.
- Flatulence - The GI tract is sluggish after birth because of hormonal changes and decreased muscle tone. Flatulence is common, especially after C-section. This is alleviated by early ambulation, turning from side to side, avoiding carbonated beverages, and taking antiflatulent medications.

Attachment/bonding

Maternal attachment processes

By the time of birth, most mothers have developed an emotional connection with her infant and demonstrate a number of typical steps in the maternal attachment process:

- Touching: The mother usually begins by lightly touching the infant's extremities with her fingertips and moving toward running the palm over the baby's trunk. This exploration of the infant can proceed very quickly (minutes) or be more tentative and take days. Early skin-to-skin contact with the infant tends to accelerate this process.
- En face positioning: The mother increases the amount of face-to-face eye contact with the infant, typically holding the infant close to her face and responding to eye contact by speaking in a sing-song high-pitched tone (baby talk).
- Responding: The mother tends to respond verbally to sounds the infant makes.

Initially, the mother may feel herself separate and distant from the child, especially if she doesn't feel an immediate bond, and the mother should be reassured that these feelings are normal.

Psychosocial Needs of the Family

Attachment/bonding

Maternal attachment phases are:

- Acquaintance - During the acquaintance period (first few days), responding helps the mother to recognize clues the child is giving about needs, such as hunger, and the mother's ability to respond to those needs strengthens the bond and helps the mother gain confidence in her parenting ability. During this time, the infant is also learning to recognize routines, such as nursing when held toward the breast.
- Mutual regulation - During this phase, which may vary in duration, the mother is learning to balance the needs of the infant against her own needs, and she may have some negative feelings, such as resenting her lack of sleep or feeling frustration with the infant's crying. The mother may be afraid to express any negative feelings, fearful that people will think she is a "bad" mother, but these feelings are normal until the mother and infant reach a mutual balance. The ability of the mother and infant to recognize each other's cues and respond to them is termed reciprocity.

Assessing maternal attachment/bonding

Assessment of maternal attachment/bonding should be done prior to discharge so that any issues and interventions can be discussed. In doing the assessment, the nurse evaluates the following:

- There should be a progression in touching and face-to-face eye contact with extended times and indications of attraction, such as verbally responding to the infant and cuddling the infant. If there is no progression, then the nurse should assess contributing environmental, cultural, and social factors that may interfere.
- The mother should show consistency in caring for the infant and seeking both knowledge about, and validation of, her infant care, adjusting care to the needs of the infant. Sensitivity to the infant's needs should be shown, such as recognizing

discomfort or hunger quickly and exhibiting pleasure at the infant's response to her efforts.

- The mother should show pleasure in the infant, expressed by calling the infant by name, noting family traits/characteristics, and showing overt happiness. If the mother shows displeasure or apathy, this may indicate poor attachment but might also indicate the mother is experiencing pain or weakness.

Paternal, sibling/family

Paternal attachment, referred to as engrossment, is in many ways similar to maternal attachment. The father may feel pride and wonderment at the child and develop a strong sense of nurturing. Early and frequent contact with the infant promotes engrossment, so the nurse should ensure that the father is not overlooked after delivery but is able to hold, touch, and respond to the child as soon as possible. Sibling and family attachment is important. Siblings should be allowed to visit the mother and infant as early as possible and encouraged to hold or care for the infant as appropriate for their ages. Siblings sometimes feel left out or overshadowed by the new infant, so it's important that the parents take time to talk to the siblings and give them attention as well. Grandparents and other family members also form attachment to the infant and should be included.

Barriers to parent infant interaction

There are many barriers to parent-infant interaction, especially with preterm infants or those with genetic disabilities/birth defects that require prolonged hospitalization or treatment. Barriers include:

- Physical separation: When the infant cannot be held or fed, when the child is transported to a different facility outside of the area, or when the mother is discharged and the infant remains hospitalized, this prevents attachment.
- Lack of clear understanding of handicaps/developmental problems: Lack of infant response is sometimes interpreted as rejection, and parents may be frightened by abnormalities.
- Attitude of medical staff: Negative attitudes may cause the parent to grieve rather than attach to the child. Staff members need to encourage the parents to become involved in the child's care and provide stimulation. Staff often needs to demonstrate care to parents, who may be intimidated by the infant's condition and medical needs.
- Environmental overload: The equipment (alarms, ventilators, monitors) and environmental constraints (no chairs) may overwhelm parents.

Education for Infant Care

Choking or gagging

Prevention is important as most choking, gagging episodes can be avoided:

- Ensure small hazardous items (pins, cotton balls) or materials (baby powder) are out of reach.
- DO NOT prop bottle for feeding.
- Burp the infant regularly during feedings (breast and bottle).
- Keep the baby in an upright position with the head elevated during feedings
- Check the nipple of bottle to ensure it is dripping and not running freely.

- If the infant is choking, secure him/her face down on the forearm tilted downward, and use the heel of the hand to thump in the mid back. Repeat as necessary. If choking does not resolve with evidence of breathing immediately, call 9-1-1 and begin CPR.

Umbilical cord

The umbilical cord changes color from grayish to brown to black as it dries and finally falls off in about 10-14 days.

- Protect the cord from moisture. Position the top of diaper so that it is folded under the cord instead of covering it.
- If the cord becomes soiled, wash with mild soap and water, rinse, and dry. (Swabbing with alcohol is still sometimes advised by physicians but is no longer recommended and may increase skin irritation.)
- Avoid covering the cord stump with clothing, which may cause irritation.
- Give the infant only sponge baths until the cord falls off in about 10-14 days.
- Report signs of infection, such as erythema, swelling, or purulent discharge.

Circumcision

The umbilical cord changes color from grayish to brown to black as it dries and finally falls off in about 10-14 days.

- Protect the cord from moisture. Position the top of diaper so that it is folded under the cord instead of covering it.
- If the cord becomes soiled, wash with mild soap and water, rinse, and dry. (Swabbing with alcohol is still sometimes advised by physicians but is no longer recommended and may increase skin irritation.)
- Avoid covering the cord stump with clothing, which may cause irritation.
- Give the infant only sponge baths until the cord falls off in about 10-14 days.
- Report signs of infection, such as erythema, swelling, or purulent discharge.
- Change the diaper immediately because urine may cause pain to the open tissue.
- Cleanse the area gently with water and pat dry.
- Apply petrolatum jelly or gauze to the incision area for about 4 days.
- Avoid using soap or commercial cleansing products, such as baby wipes, until the circumcision heals.
- Report any change, such as increased swelling, redness, temperature, or purulent discharge.

Non-circumcised penis and fontanels

The infant's foreskin is different from the adult males' and does not separate and retract until ≥5 years old.

- DO NOT attempt to retract the foreskin.
- DO NOT use cotton swabs to clean.
- Wash the penis with soap and water or just water during the routine bath.

The infant's fontanels (anterior and posterior) are covered by thick membranous tissue and should feel flat but firm.

- DO NOT be afraid to touch the fontanels or cleanse the scalp.
- Report bulging above the level of the skull as this may indicate increased intracranial pressure.
- Report a soft fontanel that sinks below the level of the skull as this may indicate dehydration.

Burping

Both breastfed and bottle fed babies require burping because they swallow air when feeding, although bottle fed babies tend to require more burping. Infants often show indications (grimacing, squirming, spitting up, or crying) that they are uncomfortable and need to burp.

- Burp the infant routinely after 2 or 3 ounces of formula or after nursing on one breast.
- Position the infant on the shoulder (with a burp cloth under the infant's head) and gently pat or rub the infant's back.
- Change to a different position if the baby doesn't burp (opposite shoulder or with the infant sitting on the lap and supported by one hand while the other hand pats or rubs the infant's back).

Positioning

Infants should be placed on their backs for sleeping. Sleeping on the stomach increases risk of sudden infant death syndrome (SIDS):

- Position the infant on the back when unattended or sleeping, but alternate the direction the head faces to prevent one side of the head from flattening (positional molding).
- Provide supervised time each day with the infant lying on the abdomen (only on firm surfaces) to strengthen the head and neck muscles and to prevent positional molding.
- Hold the infant rather than leaving him/her in carriers.
- Position the baby in the side-lying position (alternating from one side to the other), using specially designed supports to maintain the position.

Infant seat

All infants, regardless of age, must be placed properly in an infant car seat during transit. Holding an infant while the car is in motion is not safe. Car seats should be new or in very good condition and fastened according to manufacturer's guidelines to ensure safety:

- Place the car seat in the back seat and away from any side airbags.
- Always securely buckle the child into the seat.
- Face the infant seat toward the rear of the car.
- Recline the seat so that the infant's head does not fall forward.
- Place padding around (not under) the infant if the infant slouches to one side.
- Place blankets OVER the straps and buckles, not under

Bath

The infant should receive sponge baths until the cord falls off (10-14 days) and then a bath in an infant tub (NOT in an adult tub). Mild soap/shampoo intended for babies or just water alone may be used for the bath.

- Make sure the environmental temperature is warm.
- Fill tub with 2 to 3 inches of water.
- ALWAYS check water temperature to make sure it is warm and NOT HOT.
- Set hot water heaters ≤120° F to prevent inadvertent scalding.
- Support the baby during the bath with one arm under upper back to support the neck and head while holding the infant under the axilla.
- Pour water over the child with the free hand and use that hand to wash the hair and the body.
- Lift the baby from the tub and wrap in a towel to dry.
- Dry thoroughly, making sure all skin folds and crevices are dry to prevent irritation and rashes.
- Avoid use of lotions or creams.

Diaper rash

Diaper rash usually results from leaving the infant in soiled/wet diapers and/or not adequately cleansing the skin, although breastfed infants sometimes react to foods the mother has eaten. A rash may also indicate an allergic response to baby wipes or other products, such as lotions or creams. Antibiotics may cause diaper rash. In some cases, a fungal infection may occur, usually characterized by red weepy open areas. Purulent discharge may indicate infection.

- Change diapers as soon as possible when wet or soiled.
- Cleanse skin gently with water.
- Remove diaper and expose skin to air whenever possible.
- Apply barrier cream or ointment especially formulated for diaper rash to prevent or treat diaper rash.
- Contact a physician if the rash worsens and does not respond to treatment as antifungals, cortisone, or topical antibiotics may be indicated.

Fecal elimination

The first stool (meconium) is usually passed within 48 hours and is black and tarry looking. The stool then transitions to greenish as the baby nurses or takes formula, and by the third day, the stool is usually yellow or yellow-green for breastfed babies and yellow or light brown for formula-fed babies. Typically, babies have 2 to 3 stools daily by day 3 and ≥4 daily by day 5, but this may vary.

- Report abnormalities, such as bloody stools, watery stools, very hard stool, clay-colored or whitish stools, black stools (after meconium has passed), and "currant jelly" stools.
- Cleanse the skin thoroughly after defecation with mild soap and water, plain water, or unscented baby wipes.
- Examine the skin carefully for irritation.

Urinary elimination and cradle cap

Urination is estimated according to the number of wet diapers in a 24-hour period. Typically, the infant has one wet diaper the first day, 2 the next, and so on until urination stabilizes at 6 to 8 wet diapers by about day 6.

- Check the diaper frequently. Infants often urinate during or after feeding.
- Change the diapers when wet, gently cleansing skin with mild soap and water, plain water, or unscented baby wipes.

Cradle cap may appear as scaly, crusted, or flaky skin on the scalp and other parts of the face. It is not contagious and usually clears by 1 or 2 months. It is not usually a sign of poor hygiene.

- Cleanse scalp or affected areas thoroughly gently rubbing the area with a terry cloth or brushing to loosen crust or flakes.
- If the condition is persistent, try softening the crusts with olive oil, leave for 15 minutes, and then brush or gently comb to loosen crusts or flakes. Finally, wash with baby shampoo.

Special needs infant

Family involvement and education are vital for successful discharge of the special needs infant to ensure proper care. Bringing home a premature infant or one who has special needs is a daunting task for any parent. Before discharge, the following should be done:

- Educate the parents or guardian about appropriate caring methods.
- Explain how to interpret the infant's cues concerning his needs and how to respond appropriately.
- Point out the different states of alertness during their infant's sleep and wake cycles. Identify the appropriate times and methods for infant interaction.
- Coach the parents to ensure they perform each skill correctly and retain it. Observe interaction between the infant and parents in the nursery to help ensure continued wellness of the infant after discharge.
- Encourage kangaroo care immediately after birth for stable newborns because it is an excellent method to foster bonding between the neonate and the mother. For neonates who require resuscitation and medical intervention, delay kangaroo care until the neonate is stable.
- If the parents are not ready, contact Social Work for follow-up.

Assistance with feeding

<u>Breastfeeding/bottle feeding the neonate</u>

Neonates should be fed on demand. Most newborns nurse every 2 to 3 hours or bottle feed every 2 to 4 hours (8 to 12 times daily) for 20 to 40 minutes. Over time, the infant will establish a more regular feeding schedule, but this may vary widely.

- Try to recognize clues that the infant is hungry and nurse/feed before the infant begins crying frantically. Signs of hunger include licking, rooting, sucking, making fists, bringing hands to mouth, and bobbing the head.
- Stroke the infant's cheek or lower lip and a hungry infant will usually turn and try to suck the finger.

- Monitor the number of diapers per day and stools as a decrease in the average normal number may indicate dehydration and inadequate nursing/feeding.
- Observe the infant's behavior closely as some infants nurse for a while and then nap at the breast or take a break before resuming nursing/feeding. A full baby often turns away from the breast/bottle, stops sucking, or resists feeding.

Breast feeding

Positioning: During nursing, the baby should be turned toward the mother, with the face tilted up toward the mother's so they can make eye contact, and the mouth slightly below the nipple, which is pointed toward the baby's upper lip or nostrils. Holds include the following:

- Cradle: The baby is cradled in the arm on the nursing side with the arm supported by a pillow. The mother uses the opposite hand to guide the nipple and positions the infant toward her.
- Cross-cradle: The hand on the side of the breast used is free to guide the breast while the opposite arm crosses over the baby, and the hand supports the baby's head.
- Football: The infant is tucked under the arm on the nursing side with the arm supporting the baby's back and the hand the head.
- Side-lying: This position is similar to the cradle hold but the mother is reclining on her side, so there is no pressure on the abdomen. The infant is cradled by the arm on the nursing side.

Latching on and let-down: Once the infant is in position, the mother should grasp the breast using a C-hold or U-hold (to make the breast more firm) and lean toward the baby, guiding the nipple toward the infant's mouth. Brushing the nipple against the infant's mouth usually causes the infant to open the mouth and lunge toward the breast. Then, the mother guides the nipple into the infant's mouth while pulling the infant toward the breast. The infant's lower lip should be low on the areola so that the baby latches on to both the areola and the nipple. Suckling stimulates nerves in the areola and nipple, increasing production of prolactin and oxytocin, which in turn stimulate contraction of cells about the areola, causing milk to be ejected in a "let-down" (milk-ejection) reflex (sometimes associated with a tingling sensation) usually within a few minutes of nursing. It may take up to 2 weeks before let-down is efficient.

Family Planning

Contraception

Oral contraceptives

There are many methods of birth control, including the use of condoms, intrauterine devices, spermicides, and barriers, such as diaphragms, sponges, and cervical caps, but hormonal contraceptives are commonly used.

There are 2 types of oral contraceptives, but there are many different brands with differing amounts of hormones:

- Combined (estrogen [ethinyl estradiol] and progestin): These may be monophasic (constant doses), biphasic (constant estrogen but increase of progestin on day 10, or triphasic (varying doses of both).
- Progestin only: These have fewer side effects than combined forms, but can increase estrogen levels and incidence of thrombosis.

Oral contraceptives are contraindicated for those who smoke or have evidence or history of breast cancer, coronary artery disease, or elevated cholesterol because they are associated with increased risk of thrombosis. Common side effects (depending upon the particular drug) include an increase in acne and facial hair growth, weight increase, rash or itching, amenorrhea, decrease in libido, headache, nausea, ad breakthrough bleeding. Changing to a different contraceptive may alleviate symptoms.

Injectable, ring, and patch contraceptives

Newer methods of contraception include injectable, ring, and patch contraceptives. One primary advantage is that the woman does not need to remember to take pills, but risks are similar to oral contraceptives:

- NuvaRing® is a vaginal ring that in inserted vaginally and left in place about the cervix for 3 weeks. It is removed for the 4th week, during which there may be withdrawal bleeding. It is as effective as oral contraceptives.
- OrthoEvra® is a small adhesive patch that is applied to the torso, chest (excluding the breasts), arms, or thighs every week for 3 weeks and then the 4th week is patch free. It is as effective as oral contraceptives.
- DepoProvera® is injectable medroxyprogesterone acetate that is given every 13 weeks. It is contraindicated with a history of deep vein thrombosis or smoking. It may relieve symptoms of endometriosis.

Emergency contraception

Females who have had unprotected sexual intercourse, consensual or rape, are at risk for pregnancy and may desire emergency contraception. Emergency contraception inhibits ovulation and prevents pregnancy rather than aborting a pregnancy. Emergency contraceptives have been marketed for use ≤72 hours but recent studies indicate they are effective for ≤120 hours. Options include:

- Plan B or Next Choice (Levonorgestrel) - The first pill (0.75 mg) must be taken ≤120 hours (5 days) after unprotected intercourse and the second (also 0.75 mg) 12 hours later or both pills may be taken in the same initial dose.
- Plan B One-step (Levonorgestrel) - One pill (1.5 mg) only is taken ≤120 hours (5 days) after unprotected intercourse. This is now used more commonly than Plan B.
- EllaOne (Ulipristal acetate) - One pill (30 mg) is taken ≤120 hours (5 days) after unprotected intercourse. (FDA—approved for sale in US in August 2010.)

A follow-up pregnancy test should be done if the person does not menstruate within 3 weeks as the failure rate is about 1.5%. Side effects include nausea (relieved by taking medication with meals or with an antiemetic), breast tenderness, and irregular bleeding.

Contraceptive devices

Condoms and IUDs

Male and female condom: These are more effective if used with spermicide, but nonoxynol-9 (N-9) should be avoided because it interferes with protection against sexually transmitted diseases. Patients should have instruction in proper use to avoid semen leaking from the male condom. Condoms are 80-90% effective.

Intrauterine device: IUDs are usually T-shaped and are inserted through the cervix into the uterus (with the attached string palpable at the cervical opening). IUDs prevent pregnancy by causing a local inflammatory response that prevents fertilization. Some are plastic, but ParaGard® is copper, which has antisperm effects and can be left in place for up to 10 years. Mirena® releases levonorgestrel (synthetic progestin) and can be left in place for 5 years. It can be used with smokers, but there may be some side effects because of the hormone: acne, increased facial hair, and thickening of cervical mucosa. IUDs are 95-99% effective. Adverse effects of IUDs include abnormal bleeding, discharge, or infection.

Diaphragm

This round device has a flexible supporting ring and a dome-like latex cup (requiring latex allergy assessment). The concave surface (facing the cervix) is coated with spermicide before the diaphragm is inserted. The diaphragm is fitted to the individual using sized fitting rings during a pelvic exam so it seats properly below cervix and is held in place by vaginal muscles. Diaphragms range in size from 50-90 mm. They should not be placed more than 2 hours prior to intercourse because spermicide loses effectiveness. Diaphragms are left in place for at least 6 hours after intercourse (but not more than 12 hours). Each act of intercourse requires additional insertion of spermicide vaginally. The diaphragm should be washed with soap and water after use and inspected under bright light for tears or holes prior to each use. The diaphragm is 85-95% effective if used properly. Changes in weight or pregnancy can alter size requirements, so diaphragms should be refitted.

Cervical cap, sponge

Cervical cap: This latex cap is smaller than the diaphragm (22-35 mm) and more cone-shaped, and it fits about the cervix rather than below it. Like the diaphragm, it is used with spermicide. It may cause cervical irritation, so women may need Pap smears more frequently (every 3 months), but it has the advantage of being able to stay in place for up to 48 hours, but leaving in for long periods increases the risk of vaginitis and toxic shock syndrome. Cervical caps do not require additional spermicide for each act of intercourse and are 85-95% effective.

Contraceptive sponge: This is a donut-shaped spongy barrier device that is impregnated with nonoxynol-9 (N-9), so it is 85-95% effective does not protect against STDs. The sponge has a concave central indentation on one side that fits over the cervix to act as a barrier. The outside has a string for easy removal. The sponge is left in place for 6 hours after intercourse but not >30 hours.

Contraceptive practices

Coitus interruptus requires withdrawing the penis from the vagina prior to ejaculation. It is a frequently used method of birth control, especially among teenagers, but it is completely unreliable as sperm may leak prior to ejaculation. Using rhythm methods requires determining when the woman ovulates and abstinence from sex during the fertile phase, but pregnancy rates are about 40% so this method is only advised if couples are very disciplined, monitor their cycles carefully, and are willing to abstain from sex for long periods during each cycle. This method is often used because of religious restrictions against artificial birth control. Ovulation detection kits (such as Ovulindex®) are available OTC. They detect the enzyme guaiacol peroxidase in cervical mucosa. This indicates ovulation will occur in about 6 days. These kits, however, are more reliable for those attempting to become pregnant than to avoid pregnancy.

Sterilization

Vasectomy

The male's vas deferens are clipped or severed and then tied or sealed under local anesthetic. The procedure is done with one central puncture or bilateral incisions. Other birth control methods must be used for 4 to 6 weeks. It may take up to 36 ejaculations to clear remaining sperm. A sperm count is done at 6 weeks with follow-up at 6 and 12 months to check for recanalization that might restore fertility. Discomfort is usually minimal. Complications include infection, pain, hematoma, and recurrent epididymitis. Reversal techniques are 30 to 85% effective.

Tubal ligation

Tubal ligation seals the fallopian tubes to prevent conception. Various methods are available, including clipping, silicone rings, cauterization, and surgical cutting and realigning. Tubal ligation is often done during C-section or shortly after vaginal birth because the tubes are easier to isolate after pregnancy. Complications include infection, pain, perforated or burned bowel, and hemorrhage. Reversal techniques are 45 to 80% effective.

Voiding problems

Voiding problems, such as bladder retention or inability to initiate urine flow or completely empty the bladder are common after delivery because of periurethral edema. Dysuria is usually transitory. Mothers should be encouraged to try to urinate within the first hour after delivery. The mother should empty the bladder at least every 4-6 hours, and the bladder should not be palpable. Pouring warm water over the perineum or a warm shower may help relax muscles enough to promote urination. The time and amount of voiding should be recorded. Normal volume for each urination is 300 to 400 mL. Smaller amounts may indicate dehydration or incomplete bladder emptying, which may be verified by ultrasound. Repeated catheterization, >2 times in 24 hours, should be avoided. If the mother is still unable to urinate after straight catheterizations, then an indwelling catheter along with prophylactic administration of ampicillin may be considered.

Maternal Complications

Hemorrhage

Postpartal hemorrhage may be early (≤ 24 hours) or late (≤6 weeks). Normal blood loss with vaginal delivery is about 500 mL and with Caesarean about 1000 mL. Blood loss is difficult to estimate because it is mixed with amniotic fluid and mucus, and hemorrhage may be internal and not obvious on examination. Usual indications of hemorrhage, such as increased pulse, decreased blood pressure, and decreased output of urine may be delayed until about 2 L of blood loss. A significant drop in hematocrit (10 points) is indicative of hemorrhage. Early hemorrhage poses more risk of mortality than late hemorrhage. When hemorrhage is suspected, such as with steady flow of lochia rubra, then the woman's vital signs should be checked every 5 to 15 minutes and perineal pads weighed (1 mL blood weighs about 1 g). A soft boggy uterus should be massaged frequently to maintain firmness, with clots expressed. IV access should be maintained. Urinary output < 30 mL/hr should be reported to physician.

Postpartal hemorrhage

The following are causes of postpartal hemorrhage:

- Early:
    - Uterine atony: This is most common with multiple gestations, prolonged labor, labor induction, anesthesia, pre-eclampsia, and placenta previa. Uterine contractions are necessary to occlude blood flow to the placenta.
    - Genital lacerations: Lacerations may be undetected, or the episiotomy may continue to slowly ooze blood.
    - Hematomas: Trauma to blood vessels may occur, especially with pudendal anesthesia, forceps or vacuum-assisted delivery, macrosomia, and prolonged second stage of labor.
    - Inversion of uterus: This is rare but may occur with weak uterine muscles, extended labor, anesthesia, magnesium sulfate, and manual removal of placenta with excess traction. Rupture of uterus: This is also rare but can occur with previous C-section, multiparity, and induction (oxytocin). Abnormal implantation of the placenta may cause hemorrhage. Coagulopathies: DIC may occur in response to blood loss or cause blood loss.
- Late:
    - Subinvolution of the placental implantation site (failure of implantation site to shrink and heal): This leaves open tissue that may bleed.
    - Retained placental tissue: Bleeding occurs when it sloughs from the implantation site.

Infection

Metritis (Endometrial inflammation)

Metritis may result from C-section, PROM, repeated vaginal examination, fetal scalp electrode, instruments (forceps or vacuum), high-risk status of mother (e.g., drug use, smoking, or poor nutrition), pre-existing vaginal infection, and aseptic techniques. Indications include foul or scant lochia (depending on organism), uterine tenderness, temperature elevations (sawtooth pattern) 38.3 – 40°C, tachycardia, and chills.

Parametritis (Pelvic cellulitis/peritonitis)

Infection of connective tissue of broad ligament or all pelvic structures may result from bacterial invasion of cervical laceration or pelvic vein thrombophlebitis. Abscess may form. Indications include chills high fever (38.9 – 40°C), abdominal pain, uterine subinvolution, local and rebound tenderness, tachycardia, abdominal distention, nausea and vomiting.

Urinary
Urinary infection may result from birth trauma, urinary retention, and contamination (catheter). Indications include dysuria, fever, and urinary retention.

Wound
Wound infection may result from contamination of lacerations, episiotomy, and C-section incisions. Indications include erythema, local pain, purulent discharge, edema, and (rare) dehiscence.

Thrombophlebitis

Thrombophlebitis may occur in the postpartal period with indications of septic thrombophlebitis typically evident 3 to 7 days after delivery. Clot formation occurs in the vessel walls, leading to occlusion and inflammation. Fibrinolytic activity decreases during pregnancy to prevent hemorrhage occurring with delivery; however, this change can promote development of deep vein thrombosis and thrombophlebitis. Additionally, inactivity and bed rest increase risk. Coagulation usually returns to normal within about 3 days after delivery, so later onset often relates to other factors, such as a history of varicose veins. Superficial thrombophlebitis is usually evident by observable symptoms and poses less risk of clots breaking free and migrating than deep vein thrombophlebitis. Indications include the following:

- Femoral: Localized pain and swelling with edema of the leg from impaired circulation, often accompanied by fever and chills
- Pelvic: Abdominal pain, fever, and chills as well as generalized lethargy and malaise

Treatment varies depending on site and type but may include heat, anticoagulation, compression (stockings), elevation of affected limb, and limitations on activities.

Assessment of breasts

Engorgement
Production of milk sometimes outstrips demand in the first 2-3 days as the mother is starting to nurse, and the breasts become engorged (enlarged, taut, and painful). The mother should be reassured that this is fairly normal and can be relieved as new mothers may feel they should stop nursing or be afraid they are doing something wrong. Nursing frequently (every 2-3 hours) and gently massaging the breast toward the nipple during nursing should reduce engorgement. If the areola is hard, some milk should be manually expressed to soften the areola before the infant latches on. Breast pumps and heat (except in a shower) may increase engorgement. Cold compresses, acetaminophen or ibuprofen may provide relief. Engorgement usually recedes within 24 to 48 hours.

Blocked milk duct
A palpable localized lump or an area of hard swollen erythematous tissue usually indicates a blocked duct. Causes include nursing the baby in the same position or wearing constricting or poorly fitting bra. While painful, blocked ducts generally open within 24 to 48 hours with symptoms receding (as opposed to mastitis which tends to worsen). Massaging the affected area while breastfeeding, manually expressing the breast during a warm shower, applying heat to the area, and using a breast pump to completely empty the breast after feeding may all alleviate the blockage. Additionally, while breastfeeding on the

affected side, the infant should be positioned so the chin points toward the blocked area (usually using the football position). If blockage is not alleviated, blocked milk ducts may progress to mastitis.

Mastitis

If the breast becomes infected with bacteria, indications include induration, swelling, erythema, increasing fever, and acute pain. Without prompt treatment, painful abscesses may form. The infected area may be localized (sometimes appearing similar to blocked milk duct) or generalized, encompassing the whole breast. The mother may have chills and flu-like symptoms before obvious inflammation of the breast. Usually the mother becomes infected from the infant (most commonly with *Staphylococcus aureus)*, so breastfeeding does not endanger the neonate. Treatment includes antibiotics (usually penicillin G, dicloxacillin, or erythromycin) and nursing (or pumping or expressing) on the affected side to prevent abscess formation. Applying heat or massaging the breasts in a warm shower may increase circulation. Pain relief includes alternating warm and cold compresses and acetaminophen or ibuprofen.

Impact of fetal problems

Sibling responses/interventions

Siblings should be included and parents encouraged to bring them to visit and interact, as much as possible, with the neonate. If the neonate has abnormalities, this may cause stress to the siblings. Younger children may be hostile and older children ashamed. Children may feel guilty about their responses, and they may feel neglected as parents go through the stages of grief and are unable to provide the support that the siblings need. In some cases, parents may express their concern by focusing their anxiety on one of the siblings, becoming hypercritical. In these cases, staff may need to intervene by discussing observations with the parents and encouraging other family members to provide support to the siblings. Parents' groups that involve the entire family can be very helpful. Whenever possible, children should be included in education and demonstrations and encouraged to ask questions. Age-appropriate books and other materials that explain medical conditions and treatments should be available for siblings.

Steps to decrease family stress

Having a neonate admitted to the neonatal intensive care unit is a very stressful event for a family because it interrupts family interactions and the bonding process that occurs when a neonate goes home to spend time with family members. Steps to decrease family stress and encourage bonding between the neonate, mother, and family include:

- Have facilities available for families to stay close to their infant to encourage bonding.
- Maintain a play area for siblings so they are not isolated from parents.
- Encourage breastfeeding or pumping if possible.
- Permit liberal visiting times for family members.
- If it is known before birth that the infant will require critical care, let the family visit the unit and ask questions.
- Give the family contact information for support groups comprised of other parents who have children with similar illnesses.
- Encourage hands-on parental care, including kangaroo care, by both parents.

Kübler-Ross's five stages of grief

Grief is a normal response to the death or severe illness/abnormality of an infant or fetus. How a person deals with grief is very personal, and each person will grieve differently. Elisabeth Kübler-Ross identified five stages of grief in On Death and Dying (1969). A person may not go through each stage but usually goes through two of the five stages:

- Denial - The parents may be resistive to information and unable to accept that an infant is dying/impaired or believe that the infant is not theirs. They may act stunned, immobile, or detached and may be unable to respond appropriately or remember what's said, often repeatedly asking the same questions.
- Anger - As reality becomes clear, parents may react with pronounced anger, directed inward or outward. Women, especially, may blame themselves and self-anger may lead to severe depression and guilt, assuming they are to blame because of some action before or during pregnancy. Outward anger, more common in men, may be expressed as overt hostility.
- Bargaining - This involves if-then thinking (often directed at a deity): "If I go to church every day, then God will prevent this." Parents may change doctors, trying to change the outcome.
- Depression - As the parents begin to accept the loss, they may become depressed, feeling no one understands and overwhelmed with sadness. They may be tearful or crying and may withdraw or ask to be left alone.
- Acceptance - This final stage represents a form of resolution and often occurs outside of the medical environment after months. Parents are able to resume their normal activities and lose the constant preoccupation with their infant. They are able to think of the infant without severe pain. With a disabled infant, acceptance may be delayed because of daily challenges and reminders.

Impact of fetal problems

<u>Methods to support parents/family of dying neonate</u>

Parents/families of dying infants often do not receive adequate support from nursing staff who feel unprepared for dealing with parents'/families' grief and unsure of how provide comfort, but parents/families are in desperate need of this support:

- Before death:
    - Stay with the family and sit quietly, allowing them to talk, cry, or interact if they desire.
    - Avoid platitudes: "His suffering will be over soon."
    - Avoid judgmental reactions to what family members say or do and realize that anger, fear, guilt, and irrational behavior are normal responses to acute grief and stress.
    - Show caring by touching the infant and encouraging family to do the same.
    - Note: Touching hands, arms, or shoulders of family members can provide comfort, but follow clues of the family.
    - Provide referrals to support groups if available.
- Time of death:
    - Reassure family that all measures have been taken to ensure the infant's comfort.
    - Express personal feeling of loss, "She was such a sweet baby, and I'll miss her" and allow family to express feelings and memories.

- Provide information about what is happening during the dying process, explaining death rales, Cheyne-Stokes respirations, etc.
    - Alert family members to imminent death if they are not present.
    - Assist to contact clergy/spiritual advisors.
    - Respect feelings and needs of parents, siblings, and other family.
- After death:
    - Encourage parents/family members to stay with the infant as long as they wish to hold the infant and/or say goodbye.
    - Use the infant's name when talking to the family.
    - Assist them to make arrangements, such as contacting funeral home.
    - If an autopsy is required, discuss with the family and explain when it will take place.
    - If organ donation is to occur, assist the family to make arrangements.
    - Encourage family members to grieve and express emotions.
    - Send card or condolence note.

Types of grief

Anticipatory grief occurs when a child is diagnosed with a terminal illness. The parent begins to mourn over the loss of the child before he or she expires. Incongruent grief occurs when the mother and the father are "out of synch" in their grieving process, stressing their relationship. It may be due to the differences in how men and women grieve, or it may be because the woman typically bonds with the infant during the pregnancy, while the father bonds after the child is born. Delayed grief occurs when the grieving process is postponed months to years after the loss of a child. Initially, the parent may not be able to grieve appropriately, because of an inability to cope, or the pressing need to care for other family members.

Grief—Gender differences

When faced with the death of a child, men and women generally grieve differently:

- Women are often more expressive about their loss and more emotional. They are more likely to look for support from others. Men often grieve in a more solitary and cognitive manner. They are generally more oriented to fact gathering or problem-solving.
- The bond that develops between a pregnant woman and the developing fetus is unique and generally very intense. The father often forms a stronger bond after the birth of the child.

When one parent does not grieve in the same fashion as the other (incongruent grieving) this may be a source of conflict in their marriage. How a person acts on the outside is not always a true indicator of how a person is feeling on the inside.

Factors that influence a grieving family

The emotions that individuals and families experience with the loss or severe illness/disability of an infant are varied and dependent on many factors that influence grief:

- Cultural influences: Different cultures have their own practices and beliefs concerning sickness, death and dying, and varying rituals and ceremonies for processing loss.
- Family system: The family's composition, the roles of various members, and economic circumstances affect its expression of grief. A large family with extended

community support processes grief differently than a single mother living far from home.

- Siblings: The impact on other children in the family must be considered rather than concentrating on the parents alone.
- History of loss: Many diseases have a genetic component, and this may not be the first child to be affected.

Care of the mother who has had a Caesarean birth

The mother who has had a Caesarean birth has both routine postpartal and surgical needs. The mother should deep-breathe and cough (while supporting the abdomen with a pillow) and use an incentive spirometer every 2 to 4 hours during the daytime for the first few days. The mother should sit on the side of the bed within 12 hours of surgery and ambulate within 24 hours. Pain management with PCA, oral and parenteral medications, and/or relaxation techniques help the mother to ambulate and care for her infant. Epidural analgesia may continue for 24 hours after delivery and must be monitored carefully. Flatus and abdominal distention are common complaints, so the mother should avoid carbonated beverages and drinking through straws. Taking an antiflatulent (Mylicon®), turning frequently, rocking, or lying on the left side may help to expel gas. The mother should be encouraged to breastfeed but may be more comfortable sitting with the baby supported by a pillow or side-lying to prevent pressure on the incision.

Care of the high-risk mother

Diabetes mellitus

Mothers with diabetes mellitus require careful evaluation but should be encouraged to be as independent as possible in monitoring their own blood sugars and taking medications, such as insulin. Insulin requirements usually drop by 50 to 75% in the 24 hours after delivery because of the drop in hormone levels, so monitoring glucose levels and adjusting insulin dosage is important to prevent insulin reactions. The insulin needs should be reestablished over the next few days, taking in consideration diet and exercise. Diabetic mothers should be encouraged to breastfeed. Insulin needs while breastfeeding are often decreased even with increased caloric intake, so home glucose monitoring and adjustment of insulin doses must continue after discharge. With gestational diabetes, insulin can usually be discontinued after childbirth with glucose levels monitored and oral medications tried if necessary, although oral antihyperglycemic medications are contraindicated with breastfeeding.

Cardiac disease

Labor may be very taxing for the woman with cardiac disease, and she is often exhausted after birth. The postpartal period can place the mother at increased risk of complications because the changes in uterine and venous pressure increase both cardiac output and blood volume, and this can lead to decompensation within 48 hours after delivery. Vital signs must be monitored frequently and the patient positioned with the head elevated in the semi-fowlers or side-lying position. Unless precluded by medications, the mother should be encouraged to breastfeed, but the nurse may need to provide extra assistance in positioning and burping the infant to help the mother conserve energy. Adequate fluids, dietary fiber, and stool softeners prevent constipation and straining. The mother should be educated about heart disease and postpartal complications, such as hemorrhage or thrombophlebitis, which may increase the risk of heart failure.

HIV/AIDS

Mothers infected with HIV/AIDS and asymptomatic prior to pregnancy usually have no added risk for acceleration of their disease, but increased risk occurs if the CD-4 count was already low. Because about half of neonatal infections occur during birth and delivery, the HIV/AIDS mother may have an elective C-section at 38 weeks. Routine care should be provided, always using standard precautions. The mother is at increased postpartal risk of hemorrhage, urinary and endometrial/pelvic infections and poor wound healing and requires careful evaluation for complications. The mother should be educated about all aspects of her disease and the implications and need for follow-up care for both her and her infant. Mothers should be advised not to breastfeed as the virus may be transmitted through breast milk. Prior to discharge the mother should receive referrals to social agencies that can provide support.

CDC 2007 isolation guidelines—Standard precautions

The 2007 CDC isolation guidelines include both standard precautions that apply to all patients and transmission-based precautions for those with known or suspected infections, such as HIV/AIDS. Standard precautions should be utilized during treatment for all patients because all body fluids (sweat, urine, feces, blood, sputum) and non-intact skin and mucous membranes may be infected:

- Hand hygiene: Wash hands before and after each patient contact.
- Protective equipment: Use personal protective equipment (PPE), such as gloves, gowns, and masks, eye protection, and/or face shields, depending on the patient's condition and degree of exposure.
- Respiratory hygiene/Cough etiquette
  1. Educate staff, patients, family, and visitors.
  2. Post instructions (Language appropriate).
  3. Utilize source control measures, such as covering cough, disposing of tissues, using surgical mask on person coughing or on staff to prevent inhalation of droplets, and properly disposing of dressings and used equipment.
  4. Wash hands after contacting respiratory secretions.
  5. Maintain a distance of >3 feet from coughing person when possible.
- Safe injection practice: Use sterile single-use needle and syringe one time only and discard safely.

Assessments

Modified Ballard score overview

The Modified Ballard Score is used to estimate maturity and gestational age in newborn infants. It is most reliable when performed within the first 12 hours of life. The Ballard Score was modified to include evaluation of extremely premature infants with gestational ages as low as 20 weeks (score -10) and as high as 50 weeks (score 44). It scores 6 measurements of neuromuscular maturity and 6 signs of physical maturity on a scale of -1 to 4 or 5 (depending upon the category). The total score indicates the estimated gestational age for that infant:

- Neuromuscular measurements:
  - Supine posture
  - Square window (wrist)
  - Arm recoil
  - Popliteal angle
  - Scarf sign
  - Heel to ear
- Physical signs of maturity:
  - Skin characteristics
  - Presence or absence of lanugo.
  - Appearance of plantar feet surfaces.
  - Presence or absence of breast buds.
  - Eye and ear characteristics
  - Genitalia (male and female) characteristics

The Neonate

Normal

Assessments

Modified Ballard Score, 6 neuromuscular measurements:

- 1 - Observation of the infant's posture while lying supine indicates the total amount of muscle tone the infant possesses. Increased amounts of flexion of the elbows and knees correlates with increased gestational age.
- 2 - Square window test measures the resistance to stretching of extensor muscles in the infant's forearm. Increased ability for the tester to flex the infant's wrist correlates with greater gestational age.
- 3 - Arm recoil test measures the tone of the biceps muscles. Increased amount of arm recoil (flexion by the infant after the infant's arms are extended) correlates with greater gestational age.
- 4 - Popliteal angle measurement assesses the flexor tone of the knee joint. Increased resistance to flexion at the knee is associated with greater gestational age.
- 5 - Scarf sign test measures the tone of shoulder flexor muscles. Increased resistance to movement of the infant's arm across the chest is associated with greater gestational age.
- 6 - Heel to ear test measures the tone of pelvic girdle muscles. Increased resistance to movement of the infant's foot to its ear is associated with greater gestational age.

Modified Ballard Score, 6 physical signs of maturity:

- 1 - Skin: Immature infants have thin, transparent skin. The vernix caseosa begins development at the beginning of the third trimester. Dried, cracked skin occurs as this protective coating disappears after the 40th week.
- 2 - Lanugo: Fine, usually unpigmented hairs begin to appear at 24-25 weeks of gestation and thin as the neonate matures.
- 3 - Plantar surface of feet. Very immature infants have no creases on the soles of their feet. Creases develop first on the anterior portion and more mature infants will have creases over the entire sole.
- 4 - Breast buds: Fatty tissue underneath the areola that increases in size as the fetus matures.
- 5 - Ears: Increased cartilage content produces a more rigid pinna; ear recoil increases as the infant matures.
- 6:
    - Male Genitalia: The testes descend from the abdomen into the scrotum at 30 weeks of gestation and the scrotum develops rugae as the fetus matures.
    - Female Genitalia: Initially, the female fetus has a large clitoris and small labia majora. As the fetus matures, the labia majora enlarge, while the clitoris shrinks.

Preterm infants

A preterm infant is one born prior to 37 weeks gestational age. In the United States, preterm birth is the most important factor influencing infant mortality; preterm infants account for 75-80% of all neonatal morbidity and mortality. Health problems associated with premature birth include:

- Respiratory distress syndrome because of inadequate surfactant production (hyaline membrane disease)
- Hypothermia because of inadequate subcutaneous fat, small amounts of brown fat, and large skin surface area to mass ratio
- Hypoglycemia secondary to poor nutritional intake, poor nutritional stores, and increased glucose consumption associated with sepsis
- Skin trauma or infection secondary to fragile, immature skin
- Periods of apnea because of an immature respiratory center in the brain
- Intraventricular hemorrhage

The original cause of the preterm birth (such as maternal infection) may also play an integral role in the likely health problem associated with prematurity.

Infant born at 24-25 weeks

The Modified Ballard Score is used to accurately determine the gestational age of extremely premature infants. Infants born at 24-25 weeks gestational age will have:

- Skin - Very thin with visible veins. Absent or minimal vernix caseosa as it is just beginning to be secreted at 2weeks.
- Lanugo - Sparse.
- Feet - Smooth plantar surfaces or faint marks on the anterior surfaces.
- Areolae - Newly developing, breast bud not yet present.
- Eyes - Open.
- Ears - No or very limited recoil.
- Posture - Immature, indicated by limited flexion of the limbs while infant in supine position.
- Square window sign - Shows decreased flexion at the wrist of approximately 60-90°.
- Range of motion - Increased ROM (lone tone) when performing the popliteal angle, scarf sign, and heel to ear examinations.
- Arm recoil - Limited or no recoil.

Neuromuscular characteristics of a full term—40-week—infant

The following are the neuromuscular characteristics of a full term infant:

- Supine Resting Posture - Hips, knees, and arms all flexed past 90°, indicating mature muscular tone.
- Square Window - The wrist flexes to 0°, reflecting very little resistance to the extensor muscles of the wrist.
- Arm Recoil - Arms recoil past 90°. Contact between the infant's fist and face demonstrates mature tone in the biceps muscles.
- Popliteal angle - <90° knee flexion.
- Scarf Sign - The arms cannot be drawn past the ipsilateral axillary line because of the mature tone of the posterior shoulder girdle flexor muscles.

- Heel to Ear - Resistance is felt in the knee and hip when the heel is at the femoral crease because of the tone of the posterior pelvic girdle flexor muscles.

Postterm infant

Characteristics of postterm infants, born > 42 weeks gestation

Many are normal in size and appearance but some continue to grow *in utero* and weigh >4000 g and may exhibit postmaturity syndrome (about 5%), putting the infant at increased risk.

- Alert appearance (may indicated intrauterine hypoxia).
- Skin: Loose, dry, cracking, parchment-like, lacking lanugo or vernix. May have meconium staining—yellow to green (indicating recent).
- Fingernails: long (sometimes with meconium staining).
- Scalp hair: Long/thick.
- Body: long, thin (fat layers absent).
- Hypoglycemia from nutritional deprivation.
- Hypothermia because of decreased brown fat and liver glycogen
- Meconium aspiration (risk increases with oligohydramnios), increasing risk of impaired gas exchange.
- Polycythemia as response to hypoxia, increasing risk of impaired tissue perfusion.
- Seizures resulting from hypoxia.
- Cold stress (lack of fat stores).
- Congenital anomalies.

SGA

Small for gestational age (SGA) infants are those whose weight places them below the 10th percentile for their gestational age. SGA is also called dysmaturity and intrauterine growth restriction. SGA babies commonly aspirate meconium and have a low Apgar score, asphyxia, hypoglycemia, and polycythemia. Common causes of SGA include:

- Multiple gestations (twins, triplets, quadruplets).
- Constitutional SGA because both parents are small.
- Many genetic defects, such as trisomy 18 (Edwards syndrome), Down syndrome, and Turner syndrome.
- Placental malfunction or misplacement (inadequate fetal nutrition from reduced blood flow, sepsis, placenta previa, or abruptio placentae).
- Maternal disease (pre-eclampsia; high blood pressure; malnutrition; advanced diabetes mellitus; chronic kidney, heart, or respiratory disease; and anemia).
- Infections such as cytomegalovirus, toxoplasmosis, and rubella.
- Maternal tobacco, illegal drug, or alcohol use during pregnancy.
- Birth defects.

LGA

Large for gestational age (LGA) infants are those whose weight places them above the 90th percentile for their gestational age. The main pathologic cause for LGA is maternal diabetes (either gestational diabetes or diabetes mellitus). Infants exposed to elevated levels of glucose produce elevated amounts of insulin, which has an anabolic effect on the developing fetus, causing macrosomia (large body). Poor control of diabetes during pregnancy generally results in a larger infant with these common health problems:

- Delivery complications (shoulder dystocia, clavicle fracture, prolonged vaginal exit requiring use of forceps or Caesarian section, and perinatal asphyxia).
- Abnormal blood test results (hypoglycemia developing within 1-2 hours of birth, hyperbilirubinemia, hypocalcemia, hypomagnesemia, hyperviscosity [thickened blood] secondary to polycythemia [elevated platelets]).
- Jaundice.
- Feeding intolerance.
- Lethargy.
- Respiratory distress.
- Birth defects.

<u>Eyes, nose, and neck</u>
The appearance and movement of the face should be symmetric in the neonate and a number of different characteristics examined:

- Eyes - Eyes are usually blue to blue/grey with white to bluish-white sclera. Small conjunctival hemorrhages and transient strabismus or squint may be evident. Pupils should be equal and reactive. Red retinal reflex should be present. Tears are usually absent during crying. Eye blink test causes lids to close.
- Nose - Infants usually breathe through nose and should be able to breathe easily if mouth is closed. If not, the child should be examined for choanal atresia. Sense of smell is determined if the infant turns toward milk source or away from strong smells, such as alcohol.
- Neck - The infant should be able to hold head up slightly while prone, but the head lags when lifted from the supine position because of weak muscles. Neck rigidity may indicate injury to sternocleidomastoid injury.

Mouth

The mouth should be carefully examined with a gloved finger pressing against the tongue to open the mouth:

- Lips - Lips should be pink, normal-shaped, and symmetric. Thin upper lip with smooth philtrum and short palpebral fissures may indicate fetal alcohol syndrome.
- Sucking - Sucking (symmetrical) should occur if lips are touched. Asymmetric movement of the mouth may indicate injury to facial nerve.
- Gums - Gums are examined for precocious teeth and Epstein's pearls (keratin-containing cysts).
- Tongue - Tongue is examined for ridge of frenulum tissue on underside (tongue-tied) (although this is not clipped) and evidence of protrusion or hypertrophy, which can indicate various disorders, such as Down syndrome and hypothyroidism. Bluish swelling of the frenulum may indicate mucous/salivary gland retention cyst.

- Mucous membranes - Mucous membranes are examined for color and moisture, as cyanosis may indicate respiratory distress and dryness or dehydration. Excessive salivation and drooling may indicate esophageal atresia. White patches on mucous membranes/tongue indicate infection with Candida albicans.

Ears

The ears should be carefully examined for a number of different characteristics:

- Position - The insertion point of the top of the ear should be parallel to the inner and outer canthus of the eye. Low set ears may relate to a number of disorders, such as Trisomy 13 and Trisomy 18, intellectual disability, and various other disorders.
- Shape/size - Ears should be proportionate to head size and symmetric.
- Pliability - Ear should be soft and pliable. Cartilage is lacking in premature infants, and the pinna is soft. Cartilage should be firm by 38-40 weeks with 2/3 of pinna curving inward.
- Hearing - Hearing may be initially assessed by observing response to sudden loud sound. Evoked otoacoustic emissions (EOAE) and auditory brainstem response (ABR) are used for universal hearing screening.
- Tympanic membrane - Usually not examined with otoscope because of occlusion with vernix and blood after birth but should appear gray-white and vascular.

Caput succedaneum and cephalohematoma

Caput succedaneum and cephalohematoma are both examples of head molding resulting from head trauma during birthing. They can be observed during the newborn period and appear similar on physical examination because the neonate's head is swollen:

- Caput succedaneum is more common. It is a collection of fluid beneath the skin but superficial to the periosteum. It often occurs when the head presses against the dilating cervix during the birth process. Vacuum assisted deliveries also contribute to caput succedaneum. The swelling crosses suture lines. Complications are rare. Swelling usually resolves over several days.
- Cephalohematoma occurs when blood vessels between the skull and the periosteum rupture, causing a subperiosteal collection of blood. The swelling appears several hours after birth. It does not cross suture lines. Complications such as anemia or hypovolemia may occur if the amount of bleeding is large. The blood will eventually be resorbed and may cause jaundice secondary to breakdown of red blood cells.

Abdomen and rectum

The neonate's abdomen should be soft, symmetric, and rounded. A distended abdomen with engorged vessels may indicate GI abnormalities. Bowel sounds (present about an hour after birth) should be auscultated prior to palpation. The liver is usually palpable 1-2 cm below right coastal margin, and the tip of the spleen may be palpable in preterm infants only in the left lateral upper quadrant (should not extend >1 cm below the costal margin). The umbilical cord should be white or blue-white with two umbilical arteries and one umbilical vein observed and no discharge or bleeding. Presence of only one umbilical artery is associated with GI/GU congenital anomalies. Green/yellow discoloration may indicate meconium staining. The abdomen should be examined carefully for hernias while the infant is at rest and crying. The rectal area should be examined to determine if the anus is present and patent. Meconium is usually passed within 24 hours of birth. Soft swelling in the femoral area may indicate hernia or undescended testicle.

Back, spine, extremities, and musculoskeletal system
The back and spine are examined with the infant in prone position. The spine should be straight without a sacral or lumbar curve (which develops after the child begins to sit). Obvious anomalies, such as spina bifida, and indications of a pilonidal dimple, skin lesions, or tufts of hair that may indicate abnormalities should be noted. C-shaped spine may indicate spina bifida occulta; and lumbar lordosis, myelomeningocele. Extremities should be short, flexed, and able to move symmetrically through range of motion but without full extension. Arms/legs should be equal in length with feet and hands of normal size (5 digits each). Feet are flat. Hips should abduct to >60°. Cyanosis or clubbing of nails indicates cardiac anomalies; and yellow-green discoloration, meconium staining. The musculoskeletal system should be assessed for muscle tone. Maintenance of fetal position or limp tone may indicate hypoxia, CNS abnormalities, or hypoglycemia. Joint movement should be spontaneous with good muscle tone Spasticity or floppiness indicates cerebral palsy or other disorder. Jitteriness may indicate hypoglycemia or hypocalcemia.

Genitalia, male
Male genitalia should be carefully examined to determine if they are clearly male or ambiguous:

- Penis - The normal penis is usually about 2.5-3.5 cm long and 1 cm wide with the urinary meatus at the distal end in the glans. Displacement of the urethra is found with epispadias/ hypospadias. Micropenis may indicate congenital anomaly. The urethral opening should not be inflamed. The foreskin should adhere to the glans and be tight (if uncircumcised). Small white cysts are sometimes evident on the prepuce.
- Scrotum - Skin may be loose/hanging or tight/small with normal slightly darkened skin color and extensive rugae. A large scrotum should be examined by transillumination for hydrocele. If the skin is red and shiny, this may indicate orchitis. Discoloration (bruising) may be present with breech presentation.
- Testes - Testes should be descended and 1.5-2cm in diameter, but may not be in scrotum and may be retractile (moving into the upper scrotum or inguinal canal on stimulation).

Genitalia, female
Female genitalia should be assessed to determine if there are indications of gender ambiguity, as enlarged clitoris and micropenis may be similar in appearance:

- Mons - The labia majora should be symmetric and should cover the clitoris and labia minora in full-term and post-term infants although the labia minora and clitoris are exposed with preterm infants. The urinary meatus should be positioned below the clitoris. Bruising of the labia majora may be evident after vaginal birth.
- Clitoris - The clitoris is enlarged in the neonate, and bruising and edema may occur with breech birth. Hypertrophy may indicate gender abnormality.
- Vagina - The vaginal opening should be evident (0.5cm). Hymenal tag may be observed in the vagina. White or pink-tinged vaginal discharge is common for 2-4 weeks after birth. An imperforate hymen may be indicated by suprapubic mass or mass between labia majora.

Neurosensory capabilities
The neonate's crying after birth clears middle ear mucous and the eustachian tubes, and hearing becomes acute with hearing thresholds similar to adults and children. Because

hearing deficit is one of the most common congenital abnormalities, all infants should be assessed for hearing. The neonate's vision is about 10-30 times less acute than that of an adult, but the infant has peripheral vision and can fixate at 8-14 inches and can accommodate to large objects. The neonate is able to perceive shapes, colors, and faces. The neonate has a good sense of touch and reacts emotionally to tactile stimulation. The neonate has a strong sense of smell after nasal passages clear and will react to the smell of milk or turn away from strong smells. Neonates experience pain, and pain prevention/management should be part of neonatal care.

Chest and respiratory status

The neonate's chest and respiratory status should be evaluated by observation and auscultation. The chest should be symmetric and ribs flexible. The xiphoid process may protrude slightly and breasts are sometimes engorged, and the nipples may secrete small amounts of white fluid. Accessory nipples may be noted. Pulmonary function should include anterior and posterior auscultation. Abdominal movement should synchronize with respirations. Periodic breathing is common but apneic periods should be <20 seconds or they may result in cyanosis or bradycardia. The *Silverman-Anderson Index* is used to evaluate respiratory status. A score of 0 indicates normal findings and higher scores indicate respiratory distress:

- Chest/abdomen:
  - Rise together with inspiration – 0
  - Abdomen rises but upper chest lags or sinks. – 1
  - See-saw movement – 2
- Intercostals:
  - No retraction – 0
  - Minimal retraction – 1
  - Pronounced retraction – 2
- Xiphoid process:
  - No retraction – 0
  - Minimal retraction – 1
  - Pronounced retraction – 2
- Nasal flaring:
  - None – 0
  - Minimal – 1
  - Pronounced –
- Grunt (expiratory):
  - None – 0
  - Grunt heard with auscultation – 1
  - Audible grunt - 2

Skin—Pre-term, term, and postterm

Newborns' skin appearance depends on the development and thickening of their dermis, epidermis, and vernix caseosa. When skin develops during week 15 of gestation, it is initially thin and translucent. By week 20, vernix caseosa production begins. Vernix is a thick, waxy substance secreted by the sebaceous glands and mixed with sloughed-off skin cells, often described as "cheesy." The stratum corneum (protective top layer of the epidermis) develops from weeks 20-24. The epidermis continues to develop and thicken, and is able to form a water barrier by week 32. Near term, the vernix washes away and the skin becomes more wrinkled without its protection. At 24-26 weeks the skin appears translucent and red with many visible blood vessels and scant vernix. At 35-40 weeks the skin has deep cracks, no visible blood vessels, and thick vernix. At 42-44 weeks the skin is dry and peeling, no vernix, and loss of subcutaneous fat.

Skin characteristics

Skin colors vary with race, but all should be pink-tinged to some degree as skin pigmentation is slight after birth. Skin characteristics include:

- Birthmarks - Asian, African-American and other dark-skinned infants may have Mongolian spots (blue-black discoloration) on the buttocks and dorsal area. Nevus flammeus (port-wine stain) is a demarcated unraised red-purple lesion caused by capillaries below the epidermis. Nevus vasculosus (strawberry mark) is a capillary hemangioma and is a raised, demarcated dark red lesion.
- Acrocyanosis - Slight cyanosis of the hands and feet during the 2-6 hours after birth, especially if chilled. Color returns rapidly when skin blanched.
- Mottling - Common for hours to weeks after birth and may relate to prolonged periods of apnea or chilling.
- Harlequin sign - Deep color on one side of body only for 1-20 minutes. Usually transient.
- Erythema toxicum - Perifollicular lesions (1-3 mm) white or yellow with pustule appears suddenly over body (except palms and soles). Usually transient. Cause unknown.
- Milia - Small raised white spots on face from exposed sebaceous glands. Transient.

Sucking

Touching the roof of the neonate's mouth triggers sucking. The sucking reflex begins to appear at 32 weeks of gestation, but is not fully developed until 36 weeks. Premature neonates often have an immature or weak suck, and need additional patience and support to feed. Preterm neonates have difficulty coordinating sucking, swallowing and breathing simultaneously. Preterm neonates have immature neurological systems and less ability to handle external environmental stressors. Stressors include medically necessary and unavoidable frequent examinations, respiratory support from oxygen or a ventilator, administration of medications, light, noises of a busy NICU, or even oral feeds. As a neonate matures, the infants develop skills to self-soothe when stressed. Some of these skills include nonnutritive sucking:

- Sucking of hands or fingers.
- Sucking on a pacifier.
- Sucking during sleep.

Reflexes

Palmar Grasping: To elicit the reflex. stroke the infant's palm. The normal response of for the infant to grasp your finger. Grasp reflex is stronger in premature infants and fades away at 2-3 months of age. Absence indicates CNS deficit or muscle injury.

Rooting: To elicit the reflex. stroke the side of the infant's cheek. The normal response is for the infant to turn his/her head in the same direction as your touch, and opens his/her mouth to feed. Rooting reflex helps the infant find and latch onto his/her mother's breast.

Sucking: To elicit the reflex, touch the infant's mouth. The normal response is for the infant to suck. Premature infants may have an absent or weak suck reflex, as it usually develops around week 32 of gestation. Weak or absent reflex indicates CNS deficit or depression.

Moro (Startle): To elicit the reflex, make a loud sound or give the infant a gentle jolt. The normal response is for the infant to extend his/her arms, legs, and neck, and then pull back his/her arms and legs. He/she may also cry. Moro reflex disappears at 5-6 months of age. Asymmetric response indicates peripheral nerve injury, fractures (long bones, clavicle, or skull).

Blinking: To elicit the reflex flash a light at the infant's eyes. The eyelinds should close. Absence or delay may indicate cerebral palsy, hydrocephalus, and developmental delay.

Tonic neck (fencing): To elicit the reflex, with the infant supine, turn the head to one side. The extremeties should flex on the opposite side and extend on the same side. The reflex may be incomplete immediately after birth and should diminish by 4 months. Persistence >4 months may indicate neurological abnormalities.

Babinski (plantar): To elicit the reflex, stroke the lateral aspect of the sole from heel to ball of foot. The normal response is hyperextension of all toes. Persists until ≤2 years after which the toes flex.

Trunk incurvation (Galant): To elicit the reflex, with infant prone, stroke down one side of the spine (1 inch from spine). The pelvis should turn to stimulated side. Absence indicates CNS depression or lesion of spinal cord. Should disappear by 4 months.

Tongue extrusion: To elicit the reflex, touch the tip of the tongue. The neonate should push the tongue out of the mouth. Continuous or repetitive extrusion indicates CNS abnormalities or seizure activity,

Jitteriness

Jitteriness (tremor of chin and extremities) occurs in about half of neonates within the first few days of life and may persist intermittently when the child is excited or crying for ≤2 months. Jitteriness may also be present with drug withdrawal, hypoglycemia, hypocalcemia, and encephalopathy. Jitteriness must be differentiated from seizures, which may have a similar appearance. Characteristics of jitteriness include:

- Lack of ocular deviations or other abnormalities.
- Gentle restraint halts jitteriness.
- Stimulation elicits jitteriness.
- Clonic jerking has both fast and slow elements.
- Autonomic changes involving the heart rate, respirations, and blood pressure are not present.
- EEG is normal.

Jitteriness is distinct from shuddering, a 10-15 second period of fast tremors that may recur ≤100 times daily. Both jitteriness and shuddering are benign findings that require no treatment.

Normal cardiac rates

Normal cardiac rates can vary widely from one neonate to another, so it's important to understand the normal range in order to determine if the infant has an abnormal pulse. Rates will also vary depending upon whether the infant is awake, sleeping, or active. Pulse rate should be taken with a stethoscope, because the pulse may be difficult to palpate or count accurately manually. Additionally, this allows assessment for heart murmurs. Normal cardiac rates are as follows:

- Newborn infant:
    - At rest: 100-180
    - Asleep: 80-160
    - Active/sick: < 220
- 1 to 12 weeks:
    - At rest: 100-220
    - Asleep: 80-200
    - Active/sick: < 220

Monitoring of heart rate is particularly important as alterations of heart rate occur with periods of apnea. A period of apnea is usually followed by decreased heart rate as well as decrease in oxygen saturation. Respiratory rates should be monitored as well as heart rate.

Vital signs

Temperature drops rapidly (skin temperature falls 0.3°C/minute) after birth with exposure to ambient room temperature but stabilizes within 8-12 hours. Temperature is usually measured by axillary method (for 3 minutes) and ranges from 36.3°C to 37.0°C. Respiration should be 30-60 per minute. The pulse should be:

- 120-120 bpm awake
- 100 bpm asleep
- 180 bmp crying

Term infant: Normal blood pressure values include:

- Systolic-56-77 mm Hg.
- Diastolic 33-50 mm Hg.
- MAP 42-60 mm Hg.
- Hypertension: Systolic >90 and diastolic >60.

Preterm infant: In a preterm infant, systolic and diastolic values will vary depending on the gestational age and size of the infant. A preterm infant should have a mean arterial pressure that is a number matching the gestational age in weeks of that infant. For example, an infant born at 28 weeks gestation should have a MAP of 28.

- Hypertension: Systolic > 80 and diastolic >50.

Proper fit of the blood pressure cuff is imperative to obtain an accurate reading. One must measure the width of the infants arm in the area that the cuff will be applied. Once this measurement is obtained, the cuff should be approximately 25% wider than this measurement. A cuff that is too small results in BP reading too high and too large results in BP reading too low.

Appearance, weight, and measurements

- Head - Disproportionately large for body.
- Body – Long
- Extremities - Short and in flexed position. (Feet usually dorsiflexed after breech birth.)
- Hands – Clenched
- Neck - Short and chin resting on chest
- Abdomen – Prominent
- Hips – Narrow
- Chest – Rounded
- Weight - 2500-4000 g (average about 3400). Physiologic weight loss is 5-10% for full term and 155 for preterm.
- Length - 45-55 cm (average 50 cm).
- Head circumference - 32-38 cm (usually 2 cm greater than chest circumference)
- Chest circumference - 30-36 cm

Adaptations to life

Brazelton Neonatal Behavioral Assessment Scale

The Brazelton Neonatal Behavioral Assessment Scale is a multi-dimensional scale that is used to assess a neonate's state, temperament, and behavioral patterns. It includes assessment of 18 reflexes, 28 behaviors, and 6 other characteristics. It is usually completed on day 3 with an attempt to elicit the most positive response, usually when the infant is comforted and in a quiet dim room. Scoring correlates to the child's awake or sleep state. Infants are scored according to response in many areas, including:

- Habituation: Ability to diminish response to repeat stimuli.
- Visual and auditory orientation: Ability to respond to stimuli, and fixate and follow a visual object.
- Motor activity: Assessment of body tone in various activities.
- Variations: Changes in color, state, activity, alertness, and excitement during the exam.
- Self-quieting activities: Frequency and speed of self-calming activities, such as sucking on hand, putting hand to mouth, focusing on objects or sound.
- Social behaviors: Ability to cuddle, engage, and enjoy physical contact.

Routine nursing care

PKU

Phenylketonuria (PKU) is an inborn error of metabolism that results from a deficiency of the liver enzyme that changes phenylalanine to tyrosine (phenylalanine is a product that results when protein is digested). These infants are unable to digest protein. The symptoms of this disorder will show up sometime before 3 months if not caught in a screening. The first symptoms will be vomiting, poor feeding effort, and irritability. Later, if not treated, the infant will develop eczema and will have urine that smells musty. Once this condition is diagnosed, the infant must be put on a strict diet that restricts phenylalanine. Extensive family training must take place to educate the family about the diet. If the infant does not follow this diet restriction, intellectual disability will result. PKU screening within 7 days of birth is required in all 50 states.

Screening for genetic diseases

Screening of the newborn to detect genetic diseases varies somewhat from one state to another. Because about 1 in 200 newborns has chromosomal abnormalities, screening is an important tool although many birth defects are not genetic in origin, such as defects caused by maternal alcohol abuse or vitamin deficiency. Screening tests include the following:

- Biotinidase deficiency (autosomal recessive).
- Congenital adrenal hyperplasia (autosomal recessive).
- Congenital hearing loss (autosomal recessive, autosomal dominant, or mitochondrial).
- Congenital hypothyroidism (autosomal recessive or autosomal dominant).
- Cystic fibrosis (autosomal recessive).
- Galactosemia (autosomal recessive).
- Homocystinuria (autosomal recessive)
- Maple syrup urine disease (autosomal recessive).
- Medium-chain Acyl-CoA dehydrogenase (autosomal recessive).
- Phenylketonuria (autosomal recessive).
- Sickle cell disease (autosomal recessive).
- Tyrosinemia (2 types are autosomal recessive; third type is unclear).

Eye prophylaxis

Most states mandate eye prophylaxis for the newborn although a number of studies suggest that parents can safely choose to refuse this prophylaxis if the mother has had prenatal care and screening for STDs. However, most pediatricians still support prophylaxis. Medications used for prophylaxis include erythromycin eye ointment, tetracycline eye ointment, or 1% silver nitrate drops. Erythromycin is usually the drug of choice because it is active against both gonococcal and chlamydial infections. Silver nitrate is rarely used now even though it is effective because it can cause eye irritation. Ointment should be applied to the inside of the lower lids (inner canthus to outer) and the eyes then closed to help to spread the ointment. Excess ointment can be gently wiped from the eyes after 1 minute.

Autonomic response

The neonate has an autonomic response to stress, especially auditory stimuli, so neonatal units must make efforts to reduce noise levels to <45 dB. It is especially important that physical assessment take place when the baby is not stressed, so the environment should be quiet with dim lights. Typical autonomic physiological responses to noise or other stress includes:

- Lability of states.
- Increased avoidance behaviors (startle, crying).
- Increased heart rate (often initially) and bradycardia.
- Increased respiratory rate or apnea.
- Increased hypoxemia.
- Peripheral and arterial vasoconstriction with increased BP and ICP (increasing risk of intraventricular hemorrhage).

These responses cause alterations of sleep cycles with increased periods of wakefulness and agitation, interfere with habituation, and decrease approach behaviors. Additionally, infants exposed to auditory stress may develop sensorineural hearing loss and abnormal auditory processing.

Thermoregulation

Minimizing heat loss: At delivery, minimize heat loss while evaluating the newborn by following these steps:

- Dry the infant thoroughly (including hair) to minimize evaporative heat loss, and remove wet towels.
- Place a cap on the infant's head, as the head is the most significant area of heat loss.
- When the infant is to be weighed, cover the scales with a warm cloth to minimize conductive heat loss.
- Place infant in a warm environment such as:
    - Skin-to-skin contact with mother, and cover them with a warm blanket.
    - Bundled in warm blankets and given to mother to hold.
    - Underneath a preheated warmer for further evaluation or resuscitation.

Minimizing heat loss is especially important if the newborn is premature or has intrauterine growth restriction, but full term newborns also suffer if they become chilled.

Kangaroo care: Dr. Edgar Ray invented kangaroo care in the late 1970's in Bogotá, Columbia, when morbidity and mortality rates rose in his NICU, but he had limited technological resources. Kangaroo Care consists of placing the infant, after drying and warming, in minimal clothing in an upright position on the mother's bare chest between her breasts. This allows for skin-to-skin contact with the infant's head next to the mother's heart. A precipitous drop was noted in premature infant mortality after this method of care was instigated. Kangaroo care concept is to provide the neonate with closeness similar to that experienced with the mother while in the womb. Kangaroo care is maintained for as long as the neonate allows. Preterm infants attached to ventilators and IV infusions also benefit from kangaroo care. There are physiological and psychological benefits for both the neonate and the mother. Enhanced bonding between the neonate and the mother, shorter hospital stays, low cost, and decreased morbidity and mortality are all documented benefits. The benefits of kangaroo care for neonate's are the following:

- Regulation of temperature, heart and respiratory rates.
- Calming effect with decreased stress.
- Decreased episodes of apnea.
- Increased weight gain.
- Enhanced bonding with the mother.
- Fewer nosocomial infections.

The benefits to the mother of kangaroo care are:

- Enhanced bonding with the infant.
- Increased production of breast milk with higher rates of successful breastfeeding.
- Increased confidence in caring for the infant.
- Increased opportunity for teaching and assessing maternal care by nursing staff.

The benefits to the institution of kangaroo care are:

- Earlier discharge from hospital.
- Decreased morbidity and mortality (especially in developing countries).
- Decreased use of financial resources.

Thermoregulation—Skin temperature probes

Skin temperature probes are often used to monitor the temperature of the infant in an Isolette or radiant warmer. Incorrect placement of the probe can alter the reading, causing the warming device to deliver too much or too little heat. The temperature probe should not be placed over a bony area of the body or over an area where brown adipose tissue is abundant. Brown adipose tissue is abundant around the neck, the midscapular region of the back, the mediastinum and organs in the thoracic cavity, kidneys, and adrenal glands. A common probe placement area for an infant who is supine is over the liver. If the probe is not making good skin contact, it will indicate that the infant is cold, and the warmer will deliver increased amounts of heat, possibly causing hyperthermia. If the probe is underneath the infant, it may indicate an artificially warm temperature and decrease heat to the infant, causing hypothermia.

Thermoregulation—Neutral thermal environment

A neutral thermal environment (NTE) is a place in which the infant's body temperature is maintained within a normal range without alterations in metabolic rate or increased oxygen consumption (i.e., environmental temperature in which oxygen consumption and glucose consumption are lowest). Infants who are in an NTE are not utilizing energy to maintain their body temperature in the normal range. Just because an infant has a normal body temperature does not mean he/she is in an NTE. The infant may still be utilizing mechanisms, such as non-shivering thermogenesis, to maintain body temperatures, as evidenced by increased oxygen consumption and poor weight gain over time. Charts are commercially available that outline the appropriate NTE for infants based on current weight and birth weight.

Radiant warmers

Radiant warmers are devices that provide overhead heat directly to the infant. Radiant heaters provide an area for direct observation and free access to the infant, which is very useful in the initial evaluation and resuscitation (if necessary) of the newborn, or for procedures such as intubation or line placement. Radiant heat devices work best if the room temperature is kept above 25°C. Two problems related to radiant warmers include:

- Promote dehydration if an infant is placed under them for a prolonged amount of time, especially if the infant is premature.
- Risk overheating the infant or cause first-degree burns.

Temperature sensors must be appropriately placed and the infant's temperature monitored frequently to ensure the infant is not being over or under heated.

Benefits of breast milk

Breast milk is the food of choice for newborn infants. Colostrum, produced during the first few days after birth, is scant, thick, yellowish, and high in protein and antibody content. Colostrum stimulates the passage of meconium. Transitional milk (days 3-14) is thinner and white with a composition closer to mature milk. By the second week, most mothers produce 23-27 ounces of bluish-white, mature breast milk. Most neonates nurse every 1 to 3 hours for 20 to 40 minutes.

- Breast milk provides appropriate amounts of carbohydrate, protein, fat, vitamins, minerals, enzymes, and trace elements.
- It contains maternal antibodies that help bolster the infant's immature immune system.

- Breast fed babies have reduced risks of eczema, asthma, obesity, and elevated cholesterol later in life.
- Breastfeeding enhances the bond between the mother and the infant by physical contact and recognition of communication signals.
- The maternal cost is an extra 500 calories a day and extra water.
- There is no chance of causing kidney damage by mixing formula incorrectly.

Neonatal caloric requirements

The caloric needs of a neonate (pre-term or term) depend on postnatal age, activity, current weight, growth rate, thermal environment, and route of nutritional intake. Cold stress increases caloric requirements. Infants who receive parenteral nutrition need fewer calories as they do not have any fecal loss, and the nutrients are not absorbed by the gastrointestinal tract. The general requirements for adequate growth include:

- Full term infant: 100 to 120 cal/kg/day.
- Premature infants: 110 to 160 cal/kg/day.
- Infants who are recovering from surgery or have a chronic illness, such as bronchopulmonary dysplasia (BPD): ≤180 cal/kg/day.

Unfortified formulas (and most breast milk) supply 20 calories per ounce. To ingest 120 cal/kg/day, an infant needs to ingest 6 ounces/kg/day of unfortified formula or breast milk. Special formulas designed for premature infants and fortifiers that can be added to breast milk provide higher calorie contents per ounce (22 to 24 calories per ounce).

Carbohydrates, fats, and proteins

Carbohydrates: One gram of carbohydrates provides 3.4 calories. Carbohydrates should provide approximately 40-50% of total daily calories. Lactose is the predominant carbohydrate. Premature infants may be deficient in the enzyme lactase (enzyme that breaks down lactose), so premature infant formulas utilize lesser amounts of lactose, combined with glucose polymers.

Fat: One gram of fat provides 9 calories. Lipids should supply approximately 40-52% of total daily calories. Common sources of lipids include palm, soybean, coconut, and safflower oils. Premature infant formulas have a higher percentage of fat supplied as medium-chain triglycerides (MCT). MCTs can be absorbed without pancreatic lipase or bile salts that are deficient in premature infants.

Proteins: One gram of protein provides 4 calories. Proteins should provide less than 5% of total daily calories. Proteins provide amino acids that are used as building blocks for muscle and other tissues. Preterm formulas have higher protein content than term formula to help meet the increased growth requirements of preterm infants:

- Full term: 2 to 2.5 g/kg/day.
- Preterm: 3.5 to 4 g/kg/day.

Circumcision

Circumcision is surgical removal of the foreskin of the penis. Circumcision has decreased in popularity in the United States over the past 20 years, with current rates at approximately 50%. Controversies exist concerning the need for circumcision:

- Minimal advantages
    - Decreased incidence of phimosis and urinary tract infections.
    - Decreased risk for penile cancer and the contraction of sexually transmitted diseases in the adult.
- Risks
    - Bleeding.
    - Infection.
    - Pain unrelieved by anesthetic.
    - Decreased sexual sensitivity in the adult.
    - Permanent damage to the urinary tract and sex organs necessitating reconstructive surgery.

Local anesthesia or nerve block should be use to prevent pain during the procedure. If the Plastibell is used, the plastic rim stays in place 3-4 days until healing. The rim usually falls off but may be removed if still in place in 8 days. For other procedures, the glans is usually covered with petrolatum gauze for the first few days to promote healing and prevent irritation.

Respiratory problems

Birth asphyxia—Overview, mild

Birth asphyxia is the cause of many problems after birth. Birth asphyxia is defined as an event that alters the exchange of gas (oxygen and carbon dioxide). This interference with gas exchange leads to a decrease in the amount of oxygen delivered to the fetus along with an increase in the level of carbon dioxide the fetus is exposed to. This gas imbalance causes the fetus to switch from normal aerobic metabolism to anaerobic metabolism. Fetal distress results and this distress then leads to increased fetal heart rate, release of meconium into the amniotic fluid, and lowered pH. Infants experiencing birth asphyxia will often present at birth with Apgar scores that are less than 5. The following are symptoms of birth asphyxia:

- Overly alert for the first 45 minutes to one hour following birth (infants are normally sleepy after about 15 minutes following birth).
- The pupils are dilated.
- The respiratory rate and the heart rate will both be slightly increased.
- Newborn reflexes and muscle tone are normal.

Oxygen may be administered.

Complications

Respiratory problems

Birth asphyxia

Symptoms of birth asphyxia are as follows:

- Moderate
  - Hypothermia as evidenced by low body temperature.
  - Hypoglycemia as glucose stores are used up trying to supply organs needed energy.
  - Pupils are constricted.
  - Signs of respiratory distress are evident.
  - May experience seizure activity at 12-24 hours of age.
  - Lethargy (floppy infant).
  - Bradycardia.
- Severe - Note: This requires close monitoring in a NICU.
  - Pale color related to the inability of the heart to perfuse the body.
  - Cerebral edema related to apnea episodes and/or intracranial hemorrhage.

Resuscitation will vary according to the infant's condition, but warming the infant, stabilizing the glucose level, and providing oxygen or EMCO (in severe cases) may be indicated

Minimum neonatal resuscitation equipment

- Temperature
  - Thermometer.
  - Warmed drying towels, warmed swaddling blankets.
  - Radiant warmer.
  - Phototherapy equipment.
- Respiration
  - Oxygen tank and hood, flow meter, humidifier, heater, tubing, nasal prongs.
  - Bag and mask set-up (assorted sizes).
  - Laryngoscope with size 0 and 1 blades.
  - Endotracheal tubes, sizes 2.5 to 4.
  - Bulb syringe, suction catheters, sizes 6, 8, and 10 French, suction canister.
  - Cardiorespiratory monitor, oxygen analyzer.
- Fluids
  - IV needles and tubing, infusion pump, umbilical catheters (sizes 2.5 and 5 Fr).
  - Blood pressure monitor, pulse oximeter.
  - Isotonic saline,
  - D10W.
  - Sodium bicarbonate.
  - If transfusions are done here, blood drainage system, volume expander, and blood warmer.
- Drugs
  - Epinephrine.
  - Naloxone.

- Supplies & equipment
    - Various sterile surgical packs, dressings, chest tubes, scalpels, hemostat.
    - Arterial blood gas equipment and portable x-ray machine.

<u>Transient tachypnea of newborn—TTN</u>

Transient tachypnea of newborn (TTN) occurs when fluid in the lungs is not adequately absorbed after birth. The neonate usually exhibits symptoms within 36 hours of birth and the condition typically resolves within 3 days. TTN is most common in infants delivered by Caesarean section, but premature birth and mothers who smoke or have diabetes increase risk to infant. Symptoms include:

- Dyspnea (>60/min).
- Sternal retraction (mild).
- Expiratory grunt.
- Nasal flaring.
- Poor feeding (because of increased respiratory rate).

Laboratory findings are as follows:

- ABGs: Hypoxemia.
- Chest radiograph: Fluid in lungs.

Treatment:

- Monitor oxygen saturation levels.
- Provide supplemental oxygen as indicated.
- Provide intravenous fluids or nasogastric feedings is unable to take oral feedings.

<u>RDS—Symptoms and complications</u>

Respiratory distress syndrome (formerly hyaline membrane disease) occurs in premature infants and is characterized by immature development of the lungs and inadequate production of surfactant, which results in pulmonary edema, alveolar atelectasis, and injury to tissue. Symptoms include:

- Respiratory distress within hours of birth with progressive decrease in breath sounds.
- Tachypnea >60/min with increasing crackles.
- Expiratory grunt.
- Nasal flaring.
- Cyanosis.
- Paradoxical respirations.
- Decreased capillary filling time (> 3 to 4 seconds).
- Edema of face and distal extremities (hands, soles of feet).
- Oliguria.
- Tachycardia (>160 BPM).
- Hypoxemia, respiratory failure.

Laboratory findings are as follows:

- ABGs: Arterial PO2 <50 mm Hg, PCO2 ≥50, pH ≤7.25.
- Chet radiograph: Decreased volume, hazy fields, and reticulogranular density.

Complications include:

- Pulmonary air leaks.
- Bronchopulmonary dysplasia. Patent ductus arteriosus.
- Hypotension.
- Renal failure.
- Metabolic acidosis.
- Sodium imbalance (hypo or hyper).
- Hypoglycemia.
- Hypocalcemia.
- Anemia.
- Intraventricular hemorrhage.
- Seizures.
- Retinopathy of prematurity.
- Death.

RDS—Treatment

Respiratory distress syndrome is often self-limiting as the premature infant begins to produce adequate surfactant within 48 to 72 hours, but more aggressive treatment may be indicated:

- Surfactant replacement therapy:
  - Infants who are 27 to 30 weeks gestation are usually provided prophylactic surfactant replacement therapy after birth per endotracheal tube.
  - Surfactant replacement therapy for those with progressive respiratory distress is administered per inline catheter or 5Fr orogastric catheter:
  - Beractant: 4 ml/kg, repeated every 6 hours for 48 hours as needed OR
  - Poractant alfa: 2.5 ml/kg in 2 aliquots initially and 1.25 mg/kg every 12 hours as needed OR
  - Calfactant: 3 ml/kg in 2 aliquots every 12 hours to total of 3 doses.
- Other treatment:
  - Supportive treatment.
  - Supplemental oxygen.
  - CPAP via nasal prongs or endotracheal tube with assisted ventilation for hypoxemia (PaO2 <50 mm Hg) or hypercapnia (PaCO2 >60 mm Hg).
  - Manage electrolyte imbalances.
  - Manage fluid balance and provide volume replacement.
  - Dopamine or dobutamine for hypotension.
  - Pulse oximetry.

Neonatal pneumonia

Neonatal pneumonia may result from an intrauterine infection (transplacental, aspiration of meconium or infected amniotic fluid) or neonatal infection acquired during hospitalization after delivery. Premature infants are at increased risk. Common bacterial agents include *E. coli, Klebsiella, S. aureus,* group B streptococcus, *Pseudomonas*, and group A streptococci. Common viral agents include herpes simplex, cytomegalovirus, varicella, RSV, parainfluenza, enterovirus, and adenovirus. Symptoms are similar to respiratory distress and sepsis.

Symptoms include:

- Tachypnea with diminished breath sounds and rales.
- Expiratory grunting.
- Sternal retraction.
- Cyanosis.
- Hypoxemia and hypercapnia.
- Hypoglycemia.
- Shock.
- Chest x-ray: Similar to RDS.

Treatment includes the following:

- Administer antibiotics (ampicillin with an aminoglycoside initially for bacterial infection), usually for 10 to 14 days.
- Provide thermoregulation.
- Maintain blood glucose levels.
- Provide supplementary oxygen and assisted ventilation as necessary.
- Treat acidosis (respiratory and/or metabolic).
- Intravenous fluids.
- Monitor for evidence of DIC.

<u>Meconium aspiration syndrome—MAS</u>
Meconium aspiration syndrome (MAS) occurs when meconium expelled in the amniotic fluid (occurring in about 20% of pregnancies) is aspirated before, during, or after birth. Blood and amniotic fluids may be aspirated as well. Some infants may present with symptoms at birth, but sometimes symptoms are delayed for a number of hours. Symptoms are similar to TTN but more severe, and the infant appears more compromised. Symptoms include:

- Tachypnea with prolonged expirations.
- Nasal flaring and sternal retraction.
- Course crackles.
- Lethargy.
- Hypoxemia and hypercapnia.
- Cyanosis.
- Metabolic and respiratory acidosis (PaO2 decreased even with 100% oxygen).
- Hyperventilation may occur initially with hypoventilation later.
- Chest x-rays may show infiltrates, atelectasis, hypoinflated areas as well as hyperinflated areas.
- Pulmonary hypertension.
- Hypothermia.
- Hypoglycemia.
- Long-term sequelae may include airway obstruction, hyperinflation, and exercise-induced bronchospasm.

Treatment includes:

- Preventive suctioning of the oropharynx as soon as the head is delivered.
- Tracheal/bronchial suctioning to remove meconium plugs as indicated.
- Umbilical (arterial and venous) monitoring of ABGs.
- Intravenous fluids.

- Intubation, oxygen, assisted ventilation (CPAP at 5-7 cm H2O), and suctioning of the trachea for infants with respiratory distress (weak respirations, bradycardia, hypotonia).
- EMCO as indicated.
- Nitric Oxide if PPHN occurs.
- Antibiotic prophylaxis to prevent pneumonia.

Neonatal jaundice

Hyperbilirubinemia—Physiologic

Hyperbilirubinemia, excess of bilirubin in the blood, is characterized by jaundice. Hyperbilirubinemia is evaluated according to the levels of direct (conjugated) bilirubin and/or indirect (unconjugated) bilirubin:

- Direct/conjugated bilirubin levels increase with blockage of bile ducts, hepatitis or other liver damage, including drug reaction.
- Indirect/unconjugated bilirubin levels increase with anemias (such as hemolytic disorders) and transfusion reactions.

Basic types of hyperbilirubinemia are physiologic, hemolytic, breast-feeding associated, and breast milk jaundice:

- Physiologic - Common in newborns and usually benign, resulting from immature hepatic function and increased RBC hemolysis. Infants have larger red blood cells with a shorter life than adults, leading to more RBC destruction and resulting in an increased load of serum bilirubin, which the liver of the newborn cannot handle. Premature infants have an even greater physiologic jaundice as their RBCs live even shorter lives than the term infant's. Onset is usually within 24-48 hours, peaking in 72 hours for full term or 5 days for preterm infants and declining within a week. Phototherapy is the indicated treatment for total serum bilirubin ≥18 mg/dL.
- Hemolytic - Caused by blood/antigen (Rh) incompatibility with onset in first 24 hours. Preventive treatment is RhoGAM® prenatally or post-natal exchange transfusion. This type of hyperbilirubinemia may also result from ABO incompatibility, but rarely requires treatment other than phototherapy.
- Breast-feeding associated - Relates to inadequate calories during early breastfeeding with onset on 2-3 days. This slows the excretion of stool and allows bilirubin levels to rise. More frequent feeding with caloric supplements is usually sufficient, but phototherapy may be used for bilirubin 18-20 mg/dl.
- Breast milk jaundice - May result from breast milk breaking down bilirubin and its being reabsorbed in the gut. Characterized by less frequent stools and onset in 4-5th day, peaking in 10-15 days, but jaundice may persist for a number of weeks. Treatment involves discontinuing breastfeeding for 24 hours.

Neonatal jaundice

Kernicterus

Kernicterus (also called bilirubin encephalopathy) occurs when elevated serum bilirubin levels cause damage to the brain. The exact serum bilirubin level at which damage occurs is unknown. Premature infants are more susceptible to the development of kernicterus at lower serum bilirubin levels because of the immaturity of their blood-brain barrier, causing it to be more permeable to bilirubin than in full term infants. Disease processes, such as acidosis or meningitis, further lessen the competency of the blood-brain barrier. Early signs of kernicterus are divided into three phases.

- Phase I: Occurs during the first few days of life and is characterized by decreased alertness, hypotonia, and poor feeding.
- Phase II: The onset and duration of this phase is variable. Hypertonia of the extensor muscles develops. Infants may display opisthotonos (extreme hyperextension or arching of the back) and/or retrocollis (extreme arching of the neck).
- Phase III: This occurs generally after one week with the recurrence of hypotonia.

Hyperbilirubinemia—Indications for phototherapy and exchange transfusion

Phototherapy is often used to treat hyperbilirubinemia to prevent the need for exchange transfusion. For phototherapy, the infant is placed under special lights (15-20 cm above the infant) that will decrease the bilirubin levels in the blood. Indications include:

- Weight: 500 to 750 g — Serum bilirubin level: 5 to 8 mg/dL
- Weight: 751 to 1000 g — Serum bilirubin level: 6 to 10 mg/dL
- Weight: 1001-1250 g — Serum bilirubin level: 8 to 10 mg/dL
- Weight: 1251-1500 g — Serum bilirubin level: 10 to 12 mg dL

Exchange transfusions may be used for hyperbilirubinemia. Blood <72 hours old is used to maintain potassium levels. Indications include:

- Weight: 500 to 750 g — Serum bilirubin level: 12 to 15 mg/dL
- Weight: 751 to 1000 g — Serum bilirubin level: >15 mg/dL
- Weight: 1001-1250 g — Serum bilirubin level: 15-18 mg/dL
- Weight: 1251-1500 g — Serum bilirubin level: 17-20 mg/dL

There are many risks associated with exchange transfusions, including vascular complications, such as emboli or thrombosis, often related to umbilical catheters. Cardiac complications include dysrhythmias and overload, leading to arrest. Clotting disorders may result from over-heparinization (reversed with protamine sulfate). Electrolyte and glucose abnormalities as well as infection may occur.

Phototherapy

Phototherapy is commonly used to treat hyperbilirubinemia and jaundice when the total serum bilirubin (TSB) indicates the infant is at risk. Phototherapy is a treatment in which the infant is placed under special lights that decrease the bilirubin levels in the blood. The lights usually consist of one tungsten halogen lamp or 4-8 white or blue fluorescent lights and a Plexiglas® shield. The infant is placed under these lights with a protective mask covering the eyes to prevent retinal toxicity. The lights should be 15-20 cm above the infant. The lights convert bilirubin into a water-soluble compound that can be excreted by the liver into bile and eventually into the infant's stool. The success of phototherapy is directly related to the quantity of body surface area that is exposed to the lights, so the infant is clad only in a diaper to expose the most skin to the light as possible.

Hemolytic disease of the newborn

Rh (D) sensitivity may occur when an Rh-negative mother's blood contacts blood of an Rh-positive fetus, resulting in anti-D antibodies that can cross the placenta and attack the fetal Rh-positive red blood cells, resulting in hemolytic disease of the newborn (HDN). This is primarily a problem during second or subsequent pregnancies. In the fetus, hemolysis triggers increased RBC production (erythroblastosis fetalis), a form of anemia that left untreated results in severe/fatal edema (hydrops fetalis) that can cause congestive heart failure. Erythroblastosis fetalis is characterized by jaundice, fever, generalized edema, cyanosis, and hepatosplenomegaly. Hyperbilirubinemia and jaundice associated with HDN occur from RBC destruction, leading to neurological impairment (kernicterus). Treatment includes exchange transfusion in utero or after birth Hyperbilirubinemia and jaundice occur from RBC destruction, leading to neurological impairment (kernicterus). Management of fetal hemolysis may include early delivery (≥32 weeks after confirmation of pulmonary maturity if possible), with risks associated with prematurity, and intrauterine transfusion, which can cause fetal distress, hematoma, maternal-fetal hemorrhage, and fetal death (10-20%).

Hydrops fetalis

Hydrops fetalis is a condition in which the newborn is severely edematous with edema of the skin as well as in ≥2 internal compartments (ascites, pericardial and/or pleural effusion). While it may be caused by erythroblastosis fetalis related to Rh incompatibility, most cases in the United States are non-immune and often associated with other abnormalities, such as fetal hemorrhage, red blood cell production disorders, hemolytic disorders, cardiovascular abnormalities, infections (including CMV, herpes, toxoplasmosis), inborn errors of metabolism, tumors, and genetic defects. In some cases, no definitive cause can be identified. With hydrops fetalis, the production of interstitial fluid and lymphatic return are not balanced, so fluid accumulates. Mortality rates range from 60 to 90 percent, depending on underlying cause. Treatments vary but can include fetal or neonatal exchange transfusions, cardiovascular medications (digitalis, adenosine, amiodarone, procainamide), loop diuretics (furosemide), and corticosteroids. Surgical repair of underlying abnormalities or space-occupying tumors may be indicated.

Infection

<u>Congenital varicella syndrome</u>
Varicella infection (chickenpox) in the mother can affect the fetus in different ways, depending upon the time of exposure. Congenital varicella syndrome is characterized by many abnormalities, including eye abnormalities (cataracts, microphthalmia, pendular nystagmus and retinal scarring), skin abnormalities (hypertrophy and cicatrix scarring), malformation of limbs, hypoplasia of digits, retarded growth, microcephalus, abnormalities of the brain and autonomic nervous system, developmental delay, and intellectual disability. Mortality rates are high (≤50%) for those with severe defects:

- First trimester: 1% risk of congenital varicella syndrome.
- Weeks 23-20: 2% risk of congenital varicella syndrome.

- 5 days before delivery to 2 days after delivery: Neonate may develop congenital varicella (20-25%).
- 6-12 days after delivery: Neonate may contract congenital varicella but, if breast-feeding, the child may receive the mother's antibodies so the disease will be milder.

Hepatitis B, C, & E

Routine screening of all pregnant women and all newborns helps to identify those infected with hepatitis B virus (HBV). Infants are routinely immunized at discharge from hospital, at 2 months and at 6 months of age. In the case of a premature infant, the immunization schedule is started when the infant weighs 2 kg or is 2 months old. If the mother is HBV positive, surface antigen treatment of that infant should include careful bathing (wearing gloves) to remove all maternal blood and body fluids. The infant should also receive an IM injection of the hepatitis B immunoglobulin within 12 hours of birth. This immunoglobulin treatment is up to 95% effective in preventing the development of the disease in the infant. Hepatitis C is rarely transmitted to the fetus, and of those infected about 75% clear the infection by 2 years. Hepatitis E poses the greatest risk to the mother with a mortality of about 20% during pregnancy.

Enteroviruses

Enteroviruses include coxsackievirus, echovirus, and poliovirus (essentially eradicated in the United States). Most enterovirus infections (90%) in adults are asymptomatic or non-specific febrile illness with flu-like symptoms. There is no consensus regarding neonatal infections, but most researchers believe they are not acquired transplacentally but that infection occurs perineally (during delivery) or after birth (≤2 weeks) from exposure to a mother with the virus or another infected infant. Neonates are at increased risk of developing sepsis-like conditions, such as aseptic meningitis, myocarditis, and hepatitis. It may be difficult to differentiate enterovirus infection from bacterial sepsis. Because of lack of immune response, neonates <10 days are at increased risk from non-polio enteroviruses. Neonates may be lethargic, feverish, and exhibit signs of hypoperfusion (mottled skin, delay in capillary refill time, and cyanosis) and jaundice. They often feed poorly and cry inconsolably.

Toxoplasmosis

Toxoplasmosis, protozoal infection with *Toxoplasma gondii,* affects about 38% of pregnant women, who have antibodies from previous infection. About 1 in 1000 pregnant women becomes infected during pregnancy, primarily from ingesting undercooked meat or unpasteurized goat's milk, or contacting infected cat feces. Risk to the fetus is greatest if the disease occurs during the first trimester, often causing severe fetal abnormalities, such as microcephaly and hydrocephalus, or miscarriage. However, risk of fetal transmission is greatest during the 3rd trimester although 70% are born without indications of infection. Mild infection may be manifest by retinochoroiditis at birth (with other symptoms delayed). Severe infection may result in convulsions and coma from CNS abnormalities. Other abnormalities include hepatomegaly, splenomegaly, anemia, jaundice, and deafness. Maternal treatment to reduce risk of transmission to the fetus includes initially spiramycin (Rovamycine®). Pyrimethamine (Daraprim®) and sulfonamide are usually given after the 18th week. Some studies indicate treatment does not reduce the rate of mother-infant transmission but reduces the severity of abnormalities.

Group B Streptococcus—GBS

Group B *Streptococcus* is the most common neonatal bacterial infection. Many women are asymptomatic carriers. Screening of all pregnant women around 36 weeks of gestation followed by antibiotic treatment of the mother during labor can prevent neonatal infection. A mother needs at least 4 hours worth of antibiotic treatment for the infant to benefit. If an infant is born and the mother has not received the recommended treatment, the infant will often be treated with IV ampicillin and gentamicin for 10 to 14 days. If treatment is ineffective or impossible, the infant with a GBS infection that manifests in the first 24 hours after birth may develop pneumonia and/or meningitis, respiratory distress, floppiness, poor feeding, tachycardia, shock and seizures. An infant onset infection occurring at around 7 to 10 days old. Late-onset infections (usually meningitis) are generally more serious than earlier onset, and survivors often have serious damage, such as intellectual disability, quadriplegia, blindness, deafness, uncontrollable seizures, and hydrocephalus.

Guillain-Barré syndrome

Guillain-Barré syndrome (GBS) is an autoimmune disorder of the myelinated motor peripheral nervous system, often triggered by a viral gastroenteritis or *Campylobacter jejuni* infection. Congenital and neonatal GBS can occur. Diagnosis is by clinical symptoms, nerve conduction studies, and lumbar puncture, which often show increased protein with normal glucose and cell count although protein may not increase for a week or more. Needle conduction studies typically shows slowing of conduction. Symptoms may not be evident at birth but can include hypotonia with leg and arm weakness on neonatal exam. Muscle stretch reflexes may be absent. Delayed symptoms include sudden onset of acute flaccid paralysis and respiratory distress. Treatment is supportive. Infants should be hospitalized for observation and placed on ventilator support if forced vital capacity is reduced. While there is no definitive treatment, plasma exchange or IV immunoglobulin shorten the duration of symptoms.

Rubella

Women should always be vaccinated for rubella before becoming pregnant, as exposure to the virus has devastating effects on the newborn. The mother may not experience any symptoms of the disease or only mild symptoms like mild respiratory problems or rash. If the rubella exposure is during the first 4 to 5 months of pregnancy, the consequences for the infant are greater. Infants exposed to this virus *in utero* can develop a set of symptoms known as congenital rubella syndrome. This syndrome includes all or some of the following signs and symptoms:

- Intrauterine growth retardation (IUGR).
- Deafness.
- Cataracts.
- Jaundice.
- Purpura.
- Hepatosplenomegaly.
- Microcephaly.
- Chronic encephalitis.
- Cardiac defects.

Neonatal sepsis

Neonatal sepsis is a particular risk for preterm infants <1000 g and may be associated with a wide range of pathogens, both bacterial and viral. Early onset (≤72 hours) is usually related to maternal transmission and late onset (4 to 90 days) to invasive devices. Early onset sepsis most often is characterized by pneumonia and late onset by bacteremia and/or meningitis. Symptoms vary according to pathogen, onset, and primary site of infection.

- Non-specific signs of respiratory distress, CNS irritation, and metabolic disorders.
- Pneumonia: Tachypnea, sternal retraction, grunting respirations, cyanosis, and apneic periods.
- Meningitis: Stupor, irritability, indications of increasing ICP, bulging anterior fontanel (but signs may be subtle in the neonate).
- Decreased cardiac output with pulmonary hypertension, signs of shock.
- Hypo- or hyperglycemia, metabolic acidosis.
- Jaundice.
- DIC.
- Necrotizing enterocolitis.

Laboratory findings vary:

- Chest radiograph may show pneumonia.
- CT/MRI may show abscesses, obstructive hydrocephalus.
- Ultrasound may show abnormalities of ventricles and brain structures (meningitis).
- Thrombocytopenia <100,000 μL
- WBC counts may not be elevated and may not show shift to left, especially initially.
- Immature to total neutrophil ratio increased.
- Clotting abnormalities (with DIC).
- Culture and sensitivities may not show infection because of small sample size.
- CSF: Elevated WBC count and protein level and positive culture (with meningitis).
- Increased C-reactive protein.

Treatment includes:

- Intravenous antibiotics: Aminoglycoside and expanded-spectrum penicillin most common but vancomycin or oxacillin may be used for hospital-acquired infection.
- Surgical I &D of abscess.
- Ventriculoperitoneal shunt for hydronephrosis related to meningitis.
- NPO initially and then enteral feedings or TPN.
- Thermoregulation as indicated (radiant warmer, incubator).
- Maintenance of fluid balance and IV fluids as needed.
- Intubation/ventilation as needed.

Septic shock

Septic shock is most common in newborns, those >50, and those who are immunocompromised. There is no specific test to confirm a diagnosis of septic shock, so diagnosis is based on clinical findings and tests that evaluate hematologic, infectious, and metabolic states: CBC, DIC panel, electrolytes, liver function tests, BUN, creatinine, blood glucose, ABGs, urinalysis, ECG, radiographs, blood and urine cultures.

Treatment must be aggressive and includes:

- Oxygen and endotracheal intubation as necessary.
- IV access with 2-large bore catheters and central venous line.
- Rapid fluid administration of NS at 10 mL/kg, which may be repeated, or isotonic crystalloid every 5-10 minutes
- Monitoring urinary output.
- Inotropic agents (dopamine, dobutamine, norepinephrine) if no response to fluids or fluid overload.
- Empiric IV antibiotic therapy (usually with 2 broad spectrum antibiotics for both gram-positive and gram-negative bacteria) until cultures return and antibiotics may be changed.
- Hemodynamic and laboratory monitoring.
- Removing source of infection (abscess, catheter).

Septic shock is caused by toxins produced by bacteria and cytokines that the body produces in response to severe infection, resulting in a complex syndrome of disorders. Symptoms are wide-ranging:

- Initial - Hyper- or hypothermia, increased temperature (↑38ºC) with chills, tachycardia with increased pulse pressure, tachypnea, alterations in mental status (dullness), hypotension, hyperventilation with respiratory alkalosis ($PaCO2 \leq 30$ mm Hg), increased lactic acid, and unstable BP, and dehydration with increased urinary output.
- Cardiovascular - Myocardial depression and dysrhythmias.
- Respiratory - Tachypnea, respiratory failure and hypoxia.
- Renal - Acute renal failure (ARF) with decreased urinary output and increased BUN.
- Hepatic - Jaundice and liver dysfunction with increased transaminase, alkaline phosphatase and bilirubin.
- Hematologic - Mild or severe blood loss (from mucosal ulcerations), neutropenia or neutrophilia, decreased platelets, and DIC.
- Endocrine - Hyperglycemia, hypoglycemia (rare).
- Skin - Cellulitis, erysipelas, and fascitis, acrocyanotic and necrotic peripheral lesions.

<u>Bacterial meningitis</u>

Bacterial meningitis may manifest differently, depending upon the age of the infant:

- Early onset: The infant may exhibit signs of shock within 24 hours of birth with rapid progression of symptoms that include respiratory distress with episodes of apnea, hypotension, thermodysregulation, inconsolable crying, seizures, diarrhea, jaundice, and hepatomegaly.
- Late onset: Symptoms may be very nonspecific and can include weight loss, hypo- or hyperthermia, jaundice, irritability, lethargy, irregular respirations with periods of apnea. More specific signs may include increasing signs of illness, difficulty feeding with loss of suck reflex, hypotonia, posturing, weak cry, seizures, and bulging fontanels (may be a late sign). Nuchal rigidity does not usually occur with neonates but may be a late sign.

Treatment includes antibiotic therapy as indicated according to cultures and sensitivities. Initial therapy usually includes ampicillin or penicillin G and an aminoglycoside. Treatment is monitored by examination of CSF with treatment usually for two weeks after CSF becomes sterile. Kernig's sign and Brudzinski's sign are generally absent in neonates.

Ophthalmia neonatorum

Conjunctivitis is inflammation of the conjunctiva of the eye from bacteria, viruses, or chemical irritants. If infectious conjunctivitis occurs <30 days of birth, it is referred to as ophthalmia neonatorum and is commonly acquired during delivery:

- Pathogenic agents include Chlamydia trachomatis, Neisseria gonorrhea, and herpesvirus. It can also be caused by chemical irritants, such as silver nitrate (the reason it is no longer routinely used for eye prophylaxis).
- Antibiotic drops or ointment (typically erythromycin ointment) is applied to the newborns eyes to prevent conjunctivitis. Intravenous acyclovir is given to infants exposed to herpesvirus.

Untreated, gonococcal conjunctivitis usually develops in ≤5 days of birth and is characterized by purulent discharge and inflammation. It is treated with IV antibiotics (benzylpenicillin or cefotaxime). Chlamydial conjunctivitis develops at 3-14 days and is characterized by watery discharge and less inflammation that gonococcal conjunctivitis. It is treated with IV erythromycin and topical tetracycline.

Infants of diabetic mother (IDM)

Infants of diabetic mother often present with:

- Birth trauma secondary to cephalopelvic disproportion, including shoulder dislocation.
- Hypoglycemia from sudden withdrawal of maternal glucose and elevated insulin in the infant.
- Respiratory distress syndrome because elevated insulin inhibits surfactant production.
- Polycythemia (excessive red blood cell production) and hyperviscosity because elevated insulin and glucose increase the metabolic rate and oxygen consumption.
- Iron deficiency because polycythemia leaches iron from the heart and brain.
- Hyperbilirubinemia because of increased red blood cell destruction after birth.
- Cardiovascular malformations, like intraventricular hypertrophy with outflow tract obstruction, transposition of the great arteries, ventral septal defects, and coarctation of the aorta.
- Congenital malformations, like anencephaly, spina bifida, renal agenesis, and duodenal atresia.
- Electrolyte abnormalities, like hypocalcemia and hypomagnesemia.
- Macrosomia (>4000 to 4500 g) because of increased glucose transfer across the placenta.

High-Risk Infant

Acute hypoglycemia/hyperinsulinism

Acute hypoglycemia/hyperinsulinism can cause damage to the central nervous and cardiopulmonary systems, interfering with development of the brain and causing neurological impairment. Causes include:

- Persistent hyperinsulinemic hypoglycemia of infancy (PHHI) in infants of diabetic mothers, usually apparent in the first 3 months.
- Genetic defects in chromosome 11 (short arm).
- Severe infections, such as Gram-negative sepsis, endotoxic shock.
- Maternal tocolytic administration.

Symptoms are as follows:

- Blood glucose <40 mg/dL.
- Central nervous system: seizures, altered consciousness, lethargy, and poor feeding with vomiting, myoclonus, respiratory distress, diaphoresis, hypothermia, and cyanosis.
- Umbilical catheter with tip near pancreas, with glucose triggering increased production of insulin.

Treatment includes the following:

- Glucose/Glucagon administration to elevate blood glucose levels.
- Diazoxide (Hyperstat®) inhibits release of insulin.
- Somatostatin (Sandostatin®) to suppress insulin production.
- Nifedipine.
- Careful monitoring.
- Surgical removal of 85-90% of pancreas may be needed for infants to reduce insulin but poses risk of diabetes.

Fetal exposure to drugs

<u>Heroin</u>
Heroin use by the mother has a profound effect on the fetus and the neonate. Infants with prenatal heroin exposure display symmetric intrauterine growth retardation (IUGR) and are often born prematurely. Sixty to 80% of these infants will undergo neonatal abstinence syndrome (NAS). Heroin has a relatively short half-life and symptoms of NAS typically begin 48-72 hours after delivery.

Several different body systems are affected by NAS and include:

- CNS dysfunction:
    - High-pitched cry hyperactive. Reflexes increased muscle.
    - Irritability.
    - Tremors.
- GI Dysfunction:
    - Poor feeding.
    - Periods of frantic sucking or rooting.
    - Vomiting.

- Loose or watery stools.
- Vomiting.
- Miscellaneous Signs
    - Frequent yawning.
    - Sneezing multiple times.
    - Sweating.
    - Fever.
    - Tachypnea.

<u>Withdrawal symptoms</u>
Fetal exposure to drugs, such as opioids, methadone, cocaine, crack, and other recreational drugs, causes withdrawal symptoms in about 60% of infants. There are many variables, which include the type of drug and extent and duration of maternal drug use. For example, children may have withdrawal symptoms within 48 hours for cocaine, heroin, and methamphetamine exposure, but there may be delays of up to 2 -3 weeks for methadone. Short hospital stays after birth make it imperative that children at risk are identified so they can receive supportive treatment, particularly since they often feed poorly and can quickly become dehydrated and undernourished. Polydrug use makes it difficult to describe a typical profile of symptoms, but they usually include:

- Tremors.
- Irritability.
- Hypertonicity.
- High-pitched crying.
- Diarrhea.
- Dry skin.
- Seizures (in severe cases).

Treatment is supportive. Infants with opiate exposure may be given decreasing doses of opiates, such as morphine elixir, with close monitoring until the child is weaned off of the medication.

Managing symptoms of intrauterine drug exposure

The following are symptoms and interventions related to intrauterine drug exposure:

- High-pitched crying:
    - Keep room quiet with low light.
    - Swaddle the infant securely in a flexed position with the arms close to the body.
    - Hold infant close to body.
    - Rock swaddled infant slowly and rhythmically.
    - Walk with swaddled infant held close.
    - Offer pacifier, possibly with sugar solution if acceptable.
    - Give a warm bath.
    - Play soft music.
    - Place the infant in a dark room with no stimulation at all for a period of time may be effective if other methods fail.

- Inability to sleep:
    - Decrease environmental stimuli/ maintain quiet.
    - Waterbed or sheepskin.
    - Feed frequently in small amounts.
- Nasal stuffiness/sneezing:
    - Aspirate nasopharynx as needed.
    - Feed slowly and give time for rest between sucking.
    - Monitor respirations.
- Poor feeding and frantic sucking (fingers, fist):
    - Feed small frequent amounts with enteral feedings if necessary.
    - Daily weight.
    - Provide nonnutritive sucking with pacifier to relieve frantic sucking.
- Regurgitation
    - Weigh frequently and monitor fluids and electrolytes.
    - Observe for dehydration and provide IV fluids as needed.
    - Place supine with head elevated after feedings.
- Hypertonicity
    - Monitor temperature and decrease environmental temperature if infant's temperature >37.6°C.
    - Change infant's position frequently to avoid pressure sores.
    - Place on sheepskin or waterbed to prevent pressure.
- Diarrhea
    - Change diaper frequently and cleanse skin with mild soap and water. Apply skin barrier as needed.
    - Expose irritated skin to air.
- Tremor, seizures
    - Decrease environmental stimuli and handling.
    - Change position frequently.
    - Observe for scratches, blistering, or abrasions.
    - Place on sheepskin or waterbed to reduce friction and pressure.
    - Maintain patent airway and observe for apnea.
    - Monitor for hyperthermia.

Neonatal effects of C-section

Currently, about 30% of deliveries in the United States are by Caesarean section with increasing numbers of women asking for elective C-sections rather than vaginal delivery. However, C-sections pose more risk for the neonates because the lungs are not cleared of fluid as they are during labor and vaginal delivery, and if gestational age has not been accurately determined, iatrogenic prematurity may occur with associated respiratory distress. Even full-term neonates are at increased risk of transient tachypnea of newborn and persistent pulmonary hypertension. Neonates delivered by C-section typically have low APGAR scores, sometimes related to affects of anesthesia. While uncommon, the infant can also be cut during the incision. After delivery, the neonate's respiratory status must be monitored carefully, especially for the first 24 to 48 hours

Fetal exposure to AIDS/HIV

Most infants infected with AIDS/HIV acquire the infection from their mothers (vertical transmission). The perinatal transmission rate is 30% in untreated HIV positive mothers, usually acquired during delivery. Neonates are usually asymptomatic but are at risk for prematurity, low birth weight, and small for gestational age (SVA). Infants may show failure to thrive, hepatomegaly, interstitial lymphocytic pneumonia, recurrent infections, and CNS abnormalities. Optimal treatment reduces the perinatal transmission rate to as low as 1-2%:

- Antiviral therapy during the pregnancy: A reduced viral load in the mother lessens the likelihood of prenatal transmission.
- Elective caesarian section before the amniotic membranes rupture. Emergency caesarian, rupture of membranes longer than 4 hours, and the need for an episiotomy all increase the likelihood of infection during delivery.
- Antiviral medications for the neonate for the first 6 weeks of life. The first dose should be given within the first 6-12 hours after delivery.
- Avoiding breastfeeding: The risk of HIV transmission with breastfeeding is 0.7% per month of breastfeeding.

Neonatal HIV testing

The immunological status of infants with HIV positive mothers is assessed in a series of tests performed over the first two years in order to institute treatment and decrease transmission to ≤2%:

- Birth (≤24 hours): ELISA and rapid tests are used to identify those neonates who test positive at birth. Confirmatory testing is done with the neonate's blood (not cord blood), usually using DNA PCR, which is about 99% sensitive by 1 month. RNA PCR may be used for some subtypes of HIV infection.

In the United States, testing is based on identifying mothers with HIV. If the mother's status is not known, then some states require mandatory testing of the infant, but laws vary. Based on positive findings, treatment is begun within 24 hours without waiting for confirmatory test results. Breastfeeding is avoided. Subsequent testing is done at 2, 4, 12, and 18 months.

Secret Key #1 - Time is Your Greatest Enemy

Pace Yourself

Wear a watch. At the beginning of the test, check the time (or start a chronometer on your watch to count the minutes), and check the time after every few questions to make sure you are "on schedule."

If you are forced to speed up, do it efficiently. Usually one or more answer choices can be eliminated without too much difficulty. Above all, don't panic. Don't speed up and just begin guessing at random choices. By pacing yourself, and continually monitoring your progress against your watch, you will always know exactly how far ahead or behind you are with your available time. If you find that you are one minute behind on the test, don't skip one question without spending any time on it, just to catch back up. Take 15 fewer seconds on the next four questions, and after four questions you'll have caught back up. Once you catch back up, you can continue working each problem at your normal pace.

Furthermore, don't dwell on the problems that you were rushed on. If a problem was taking up too much time and you made a hurried guess, it must be difficult. The difficult questions are the ones you are most likely to miss anyway, so it isn't a big loss. It is better to end with more time than you need than to run out of time.

Lastly, sometimes it is beneficial to slow down if you are constantly getting ahead of time. You are always more likely to catch a careless mistake by working more slowly than quickly, and among very high-scoring test takers (those who are likely to have lots of time left over), careless errors affect the score more than mastery of material.

Secret Key #2 - Guessing is not Guesswork

You probably know that guessing is a good idea - unlike other standardized tests, there is no penalty for getting a wrong answer. Even if you have no idea about a question, you still have a 20-25% chance of getting it right.

Most test takers do not understand the impact that proper guessing can have on their score. Unless you score extremely high, guessing will significantly contribute to your final score.

Monkeys Take the Test

What most test takers don't realize is that to insure that 20-25% chance, you have to guess randomly. If you put 20 monkeys in a room to take this test, assuming they answered once per question and behaved themselves, on average they would get 20-25% of the questions correct. Put 20 test takers in the room, and the average will be much lower among guessed questions. Why?

1. The test writers intentionally write deceptive answer choices that "look" right. A test taker has no idea about a question, so picks the "best looking" answer, which is often

wrong. The monkey has no idea what looks good and what doesn't, so will consistently be lucky about 20-25% of the time.

2. Test takers will eliminate answer choices from the guessing pool based on a hunch or intuition. Simple but correct answers often get excluded, leaving a 0% chance of being correct. The monkey has no clue, and often gets lucky with the best choice.

This is why the process of elimination endorsed by most test courses is flawed and detrimental to your performance- test takers don't guess, they make an ignorant stab in the dark that is usually worse than random.

$5 Challenge

Let me introduce one of the most valuable ideas of this course- the $5 challenge:

You only mark your "best guess" if you are willing to bet $5 on it.
You only eliminate choices from guessing if you are willing to bet $5 on it.

Why $5? Five dollars is an amount of money that is small yet not insignificant, and can really add up fast (20 questions could cost you $100). Likewise, each answer choice on one question of the test will have a small impact on your overall score, but it can really add up to a lot of points in the end.

The process of elimination IS valuable. The following shows your chance of guessing it right:

If you eliminate wrong answer choices until only this many remain:	Chance of getting it correct:
1	100%
2	50%
3	33%

However, if you accidentally eliminate the right answer or go on a hunch for an incorrect answer, your chances drop dramatically: to 0%. By guessing among all the answer choices, you are GUARANTEED to have a shot at the right answer.

That's why the $5 test is so valuable- if you give up the advantage and safety of a pure guess, it had better be worth the risk.

What we still haven't covered is how to be sure that whatever guess you make is truly random. Here's the easiest way:

Always pick the first answer choice among those remaining.

Such a technique means that you have decided, **before you see a single test question**, exactly how you are going to guess- and since the order of choices tells you nothing about which one is correct, this guessing technique is perfectly random.

This section is not meant to scare you away from making educated guesses or eliminating choices- you just need to define when a choice is worth eliminating. The $5 test, along with a pre-defined random guessing strategy, is the best way to make sure you reap all of the benefits of guessing.

Secret Key #3 - Practice Smarter, Not Harder

Many test takers delay the test preparation process because they dread the awful amounts of practice time they think necessary to succeed on the test. We have refined an effective method that will take you only a fraction of the time.

There are a number of "obstacles" in your way to succeed. Among these are answering questions, finishing in time, and mastering test-taking strategies. All must be executed on the day of the test at peak performance, or your score will suffer. The test is a mental marathon that has a large impact on your future.

Just like a marathon runner, it is important to work your way up to the full challenge. So first you just worry about questions, and then time, and finally strategy:

Success Strategy

1. Find a good source for practice tests.
2. If you are willing to make a larger time investment, consider using more than one study guide- often the different approaches of multiple authors will help you "get" difficult concepts.
3. Take a practice test with no time constraints, with all study helps "open book." Take your time with questions and focus on applying strategies.
4. Take a practice test with time constraints, with all guides "open book."
5. Take a final practice test with no open material and time limits

If you have time to take more practice tests, just repeat step 5. By gradually exposing yourself to the full rigors of the test environment, you will condition your mind to the stress of test day and maximize your success.

Secret Key #4 - Prepare, Don't Procrastinate

Let me state an obvious fact: if you take the test three times, you will get three different scores. This is due to the way you feel on test day, the level of preparedness you have, and, despite the test writers' claims to the contrary, some tests WILL be easier for you than others.

Since your future depends so much on your score, you should maximize your chances of success. In order to maximize the likelihood of success, you've got to prepare in advance. This means taking practice tests and spending time learning the information and test taking strategies you will need to succeed.

Never take the test as a "practice" test, expecting that you can just take it again if you need to. Feel free to take sample tests on your own, but when you go to take the official test, be prepared, be focused, and do your best the first time!

Secret Key #5 - Test Yourself

Everyone knows that time is money. There is no need to spend too much of your time or too little of your time preparing for the test. You should only spend as much of your precious time preparing as is necessary for you to get the score you need.

Once you have taken a practice test under real conditions of time constraints, then you will know if you are ready for the test or not.

If you have scored extremely high the first time that you take the practice test, then there is not much point in spending countless hours studying. You are already there.

Benchmark your abilities by retaking practice tests and seeing how much you have improved. Once you score high enough to guarantee success, then you are ready.

If you have scored well below where you need, then knuckle down and begin studying in earnest. Check your improvement regularly through the use of practice tests under real conditions. Above all, don't worry, panic, or give up. The key is perseverance!

Then, when you go to take the test, remain confident and remember how well you did on the practice tests. If you can score high enough on a practice test, then you can do the same on the real thing.

General Strategies

The most important thing you can do is to ignore your fears and jump into the test immediately- do not be overwhelmed by any strange-sounding terms. You have to jump into the test like jumping into a pool- all at once is the easiest way.

Make Predictions

As you read and understand the question, try to guess what the answer will be. Remember that several of the answer choices are wrong, and once you begin reading them, your mind will immediately become cluttered with answer choices designed to throw you off. Your mind is typically the most focused immediately after you have read the question and digested its contents. If you can, try to predict what the correct answer will be. You may be surprised at what you can predict.

Quickly scan the choices and see if your prediction is in the listed answer choices. If it is, then you can be quite confident that you have the right answer. It still won't hurt to check the other answer choices, but most of the time, you've got it!

Answer the Question

It may seem obvious to only pick answer choices that answer the question, but the test writers can create some excellent answer choices that are wrong. Don't pick an answer just because it sounds right, or you believe it to be true. It MUST answer the question. Once you've made your selection, always go back and check it against the question and make sure that you didn't misread the question, and the answer choice does answer the question posed.

Benchmark

After you read the first answer choice, decide if you think it sounds correct or not. If it doesn't, move on to the next answer choice. If it does, mentally mark that answer choice. This doesn't mean that you've definitely selected it as your answer choice, it just means that it's the best you've seen thus far. Go ahead and read the next choice. If the next choice is worse than the one you've already selected, keep going to the next answer choice. If the next choice is better than the choice you've already selected, mentally mark the new answer choice as your best guess.

The first answer choice that you select becomes your standard. Every other answer choice must be benchmarked against that standard. That choice is correct until proven otherwise by another answer choice beating it out. Once you've decided that no other answer choice seems as good, do one final check to ensure that your answer choice answers the question posed.

Valid Information

Don't discount any of the information provided in the question. Every piece of information may be necessary to determine the correct answer. None of the information in the question is there to throw you off (while the answer choices will certainly have information to throw you off). If two seemingly unrelated topics are discussed, don't ignore either. You can be confident there is a relationship, or it wouldn't be included in the question, and you are probably going to have to determine what is that relationship to find the answer.

Avoid "Fact Traps"

Don't get distracted by a choice that is factually true. Your search is for the answer that answers the question. Stay focused and don't fall for an answer that is true but incorrect. Always go back to the question and make sure you're choosing an answer that actually answers the question and is not just a true statement. An answer can be factually correct, but it MUST answer the question asked. Additionally, two answers can both be seemingly correct, so be sure to read all of the answer choices, and make sure that you get the one that BEST answers the question.

Milk the Question

Some of the questions may throw you completely off. They might deal with a subject you have not been exposed to, or one that you haven't reviewed in years. While your lack of knowledge about the subject will be a hindrance, the question itself can give you many clues that will help you find the correct answer. Read the question carefully and look for clues. Watch particularly for adjectives and nouns describing difficult terms or words that you don't recognize. Regardless of if you completely understand a word or not, replacing it with a synonym either provided or one you more familiar with may help you to understand what the questions are asking. Rather than wracking your mind about specific detailed information concerning a difficult term or word, try to use mental substitutes that are easier to understand.

The Trap of Familiarity

Don't just choose a word because you recognize it. On difficult questions, you may not recognize a number of words in the answer choices. The test writers don't put "make-believe" words on the test; so don't think that just because you only recognize all the words in one answer choice means that answer choice must be correct. If you only recognize words in one answer choice, then focus on that one. Is it correct? Try your best to determine if it is correct. If it is, that is great, but if it doesn't, eliminate it. Each word and answer choice you eliminate increases your chances of getting the question correct, even if you then have to guess among the unfamiliar choices.

Eliminate Answers

Eliminate choices as soon as you realize they are wrong. But be careful! Make sure you consider all of the possible answer choices. Just because one appears right, doesn't mean that the next one won't be even better! The test writers will usually put more than one good answer choice for every question, so read all of them. Don't worry if you are stuck between two that seem right. By getting down to just two remaining possible choices, your odds are now 50/50. Rather than wasting too much time, play the odds. You are guessing, but guessing wisely, because you've been able to knock out some of the answer choices that you know are wrong. If you are eliminating choices and realize that the last answer choice you are left with is also obviously wrong, don't panic. Start over and consider each choice again. There may easily be something that you missed the first time and will realize on the second pass.

Tough Questions

If you are stumped on a problem or it appears too hard or too difficult, don't waste time. Move on! Remember though, if you can quickly check for obviously incorrect answer choices, your chances of guessing correctly are greatly improved. Before you completely give up, at least try to knock out a couple of possible answers. Eliminate what you can and then guess at the remaining answer choices before moving on.

Brainstorm

If you get stuck on a difficult question, spend a few seconds quickly brainstorming. Run through the complete list of possible answer choices. Look at each choice and ask yourself, "Could this answer the question satisfactorily?" Go through each answer choice and consider it independently of the other. By systematically going through all possibilities, you may find something that you would otherwise overlook. Remember that when you get stuck, it's important to try to keep moving.

Read Carefully

Understand the problem. Read the question and answer choices carefully. Don't miss the question because you misread the terms. You have plenty of time to read each question thoroughly and make sure you understand what is being asked. Yet a happy medium must be attained, so don't waste too much time. You must read carefully, but efficiently.

Face Value

When in doubt, use common sense. Always accept the situation in the problem at face value. Don't read too much into it. These problems will not require you to make huge leaps of logic. The test writers aren't trying to throw you off with a cheap trick. If you have to go beyond creativity and make a leap of logic in order to have an answer choice answer the question, then you should look at the other answer choices. Don't overcomplicate the problem by creating theoretical relationships or explanations that will warp time or space. These are normal problems rooted in reality. It's just that the applicable relationship or explanation may not be readily apparent and you have to figure things out. Use your common sense to interpret anything that isn't clear.

Prefixes

If you're having trouble with a word in the question or answer choices, try dissecting it. Take advantage of every clue that the word might include. Prefixes and suffixes can be a huge help. Usually they allow you to determine a basic meaning. Pre- means before, post- means after, pro - is positive, de- is negative. From these prefixes and suffixes, you can get an idea of the general meaning of the word and try to put it into context. Beware though of any traps. Just because con is the opposite of pro, doesn't necessarily mean congress is the opposite of progress!

Hedge Phrases

Watch out for critical "hedge" phrases, such as likely, may, can, will often, sometimes, often, almost, mostly, usually, generally, rarely, sometimes. Question writers insert these hedge phrases to cover every possibility. Often an answer choice will be wrong simply because it leaves no room for exception. Avoid answer choices that have definitive words like "exactly," and "always".

Switchback Words

Stay alert for "switchbacks". These are the words and phrases frequently used to alert you to shifts in thought. The most common switchback word is "but". Others include although, however, nevertheless, on the other hand, even though, while, in spite of, despite, regardless of.

New Information

Correct answer choices will rarely have completely new information included. Answer choices typically are straightforward reflections of the material asked about and will directly relate to the question. If a new piece of information is included in an answer choice that doesn't even seem to relate to the topic being asked about, then that answer choice is likely incorrect. All of the information needed to answer the question is usually provided for you, and so you should not have to make guesses that are unsupported or choose answer choices that require unknown information that cannot be reasoned on its own.

Time Management

On technical questions, don't get lost on the technical terms. Don't spend too much time on any one question. If you don't know what a term means, then since you don't have a dictionary, odds are you aren't going to get much further. You should immediately recognize terms as whether or not you know them. If you don't, work with the other clues that you have, the other answer choices and terms provided, but don't waste too much time trying to figure out a difficult term.

Contextual Clues

Look for contextual clues. An answer can be right but not correct. The contextual clues will help you find the answer that is most right and is correct. Understand the context in which a phrase or statement is made. This will help you make important distinctions.

Don't Panic

Panicking will not answer any questions for you. Therefore, it isn't helpful. When you first see the question, if your mind goes blank, take a deep breath. Force yourself to mechanically go through the steps of solving the problem and using the strategies you've learned.

Pace Yourself

Don't get clock fever. It's easy to be overwhelmed when you're looking at a page full of questions, your mind is full of random thoughts and feeling confused, and the clock is ticking down faster than you would like. Calm down and maintain the pace that you have set for yourself. As long as you are on track by monitoring your pace, you are guaranteed to have enough time for yourself. When you get to the last few minutes of the test, it may seem like you won't have enough time left, but if you only have as many questions as you should have left at that point, then you're right on track!

Answer Selection

The best way to pick an answer choice is to eliminate all of those that are wrong, until only one is left and confirm that is the correct answer. Sometimes though, an answer choice may immediately look right. Be careful! Take a second to make sure that the other choices are not equally obvious. Don't make a hasty mistake. There are only two times that you should stop before checking other answers. First is when you are positive that the answer choice you have selected is correct. Second is when time is almost out and you have to make a quick guess!

Check Your Work

Since you will probably not know every term listed and the answer to every question, it is important that you get credit for the ones that you do know. Don't miss any questions through careless mistakes. If at all possible, try to take a second to look back over your answer selection and make sure you've selected the correct answer choice and haven't made a costly careless mistake (such as marking an answer choice that you didn't mean to mark). This quick double check should more than pay for itself in caught mistakes for the time it costs.

Beware of Directly Quoted Answers

Sometimes an answer choice will repeat word for word a portion of the question or reference section. However, beware of such exact duplication – it may be a trap! More than likely, the correct choice will paraphrase or summarize a point, rather than being exactly the same wording.

Slang

Scientific sounding answers are better than slang ones. An answer choice that begins "To compare the outcomes…" is much more likely to be correct than one that begins "Because some people insisted…"

Extreme Statements

Avoid wild answers that throw out highly controversial ideas that are proclaimed as established fact. An answer choice that states the "process should be used in certain situations, if…" is much more likely to be correct than one that states the "process should be discontinued completely." The first is a calm rational statement and doesn't even make a definitive, uncompromising stance, using a hedge word "if" to provide wiggle room, whereas the second choice is a radical idea and far more extreme.

Answer Choice Families

When you have two or more answer choices that are direct opposites or parallels, one of them is usually the correct answer. For instance, if one answer choice states "x increases" and another answer choice states "x decreases" or "y increases," then those two or three answer choices are very similar in construction and fall into the same family of answer choices. A family of answer choices is when two or three answer choices are very similar in construction, and yet often have a directly opposite meaning. Usually the correct answer choice will be in that family of answer choices. The "odd man out" or answer choice that doesn't seem to fit the parallel construction of the other answer choices is more likely to be incorrect.

Special Report: How to Overcome Test Anxiety

The very nature of tests caters to some level of anxiety, nervousness or tension, just as we feel for any important event that occurs in our lives. A little bit of anxiety or nervousness can be a good thing. It helps us with motivation, and makes achievement just that much sweeter. However, too much anxiety can be a problem; especially if it hinders our ability to function and perform.

"Test anxiety," is the term that refers to the emotional reactions that some test-takers experience when faced with a test or exam. Having a fear of testing and exams is based upon a rational fear, since the test-taker's performance can shape the course of an academic career. Nevertheless, experiencing excessive fear of examinations will only interfere with the test-takers ability to perform, and his/her chances to be successful.

There are a large variety of causes that can contribute to the development and sensation of test anxiety. These include, but are not limited to lack of performance and worrying about issues surrounding the test.

Lack of Preparation

Lack of preparation can be identified by the following behaviors or situations:

Not scheduling enough time to study, and therefore cramming the night before the test or exam
Managing time poorly, to create the sensation that there is not enough time to do everything
Failing to organize the text information in advance, so that the study material consists of the entire text and not simply the pertinent information
Poor overall studying habits

Worrying, on the other hand, can be related to both the test taker, or many other factors around him/her that will be affected by the results of the test. These include worrying about:

Previous performances on similar exams, or exams in general
How friends and other students are achieving
The negative consequences that will result from a poor grade or failure

There are three primary elements to test anxiety. Physical components, which involve the same typical bodily reactions as those to acute anxiety (to be discussed below). Emotional factors have to do with fear or panic. Mental or cognitive issues concerning attention spans and memory abilities.

Physical Signals

There are many different symptoms of test anxiety, and these are not limited to mental and emotional strain. Frequently there are a range of physical signals that will let a test taker know that he/she is suffering from test anxiety. These bodily changes can include the following:

Perspiring
Sweaty palms
Wet, trembling hands
Nausea
Dry mouth
A knot in the stomach
Headache
Faintness
Muscle tension
Aching shoulders, back and neck
Rapid heart beat
Feeling too hot/cold

To recognize the sensation of test anxiety, a test-taker should monitor him/herself for the following sensations:

The physical distress symptoms as listed above
Emotional sensitivity, expressing emotional feelings such as the need to cry or laugh too much, or a sensation of anger or helplessness
A decreased ability to think, causing the test-taker to blank out or have racing thoughts that are hard to organize or control.

Though most students will feel some level of anxiety when faced with a test or exam, the majority can cope with that anxiety and maintain it at a manageable level. However, those who cannot are faced with a very real and very serious condition, which can and should be controlled for the immeasurable benefit of this sufferer.

Naturally, these sensations lead to negative results for the testing experience. The most common effects of test anxiety have to do with nervousness and mental blocking.

Nervousness

Nervousness can appear in several different levels:

The test-taker's difficulty, or even inability to read and understand the questions on the test
The difficulty or inability to organize thoughts to a coherent form
The difficulty or inability to recall key words and concepts relating to the testing questions (especially essays)
The receipt of poor grades on a test, though the test material was well known by the test taker

Conversely, a person may also experience mental blocking, which involves:

Blanking out on test questions
Only remembering the correct answers to the questions when the test has already finished.

Fortunately for test anxiety sufferers, beating these feelings, to a large degree, has to do with proper preparation. When a test taker has a feeling of preparedness, then anxiety will be dramatically lessened.

The first step to resolving anxiety issues is to distinguish which of the two types of anxiety are being suffered. If the anxiety is a direct result of a lack of preparation, this should be considered a normal reaction, and the anxiety level (as opposed to the test results) shouldn't be anything to worry about. However, if, when adequately prepared, the test-taker still panics, blanks out, or seems to overreact, this is not a fully rational reaction. While this can be considered normal too, there are many ways to combat and overcome these effects.

Remember that anxiety cannot be entirely eliminated, however, there are ways to minimize it, to make the anxiety easier to manage. Preparation is one of the best ways to minimize test anxiety. Therefore the following techniques are wise in order to best fight off any anxiety that may want to build.

To begin with, try to avoid cramming before a test, whenever it is possible. By trying to memorize an entire term's worth of information in one day, you'll be shocking your system, and not giving yourself a very good chance to absorb the information. This is an easy path to anxiety, so for those who suffer from test anxiety, cramming should not even be considered an option.

Instead of cramming, work throughout the semester to combine all of the material which is presented throughout the semester, and work on it gradually as the course goes by, making sure to master the main concepts first, leaving minor details for a week or so before the test.

To study for the upcoming exam, be sure to pose questions that may be on the examination, to gauge the ability to answer them by integrating the ideas from your texts, notes and lectures, as well as any supplementary readings.

If it is truly impossible to cover all of the information that was covered in that particular term, concentrate on the most important portions, that can be covered very well. Learn these concepts as best as possible, so that when the test comes, a goal can be made to use these concepts as presentations of your knowledge.

In addition to study habits, changes in attitude are critical to beating a struggle with test anxiety. In fact, an improvement of the perspective over the entire test-taking experience can actually help a test taker to enjoy studying and therefore improve the overall experience. Be certain not to overemphasize the significance of the grade - know that the result of the test is neither a reflection of self worth, nor is it a measure of intelligence; one grade will not predict a person's future success.

To improve an overall testing outlook, the following steps should be tried:

Keeping in mind that the most reasonable expectation for taking a test is to expect to try to demonstrate as much of what you know as you possibly can.
Reminding ourselves that a test is only one test; this is not the only one, and there will be others.
The thought of thinking of oneself in an irrational, all-or-nothing term should be avoided at all costs.
A reward should be designated for after the test, so there's something to look forward to. Whether it be going to a movie, going out to eat, or simply visiting friends, schedule it in advance, and do it no matter what result is expected on the exam.

Test-takers should also keep in mind that the basics are some of the most important things, even beyond anti-anxiety techniques and studying. Never neglect the basic social, emotional and biological needs, in order to try to absorb information. In order to best achieve, these three factors must be held as just as important as the studying itself.

Study Steps

Remember the following important steps for studying:

Maintain healthy nutrition and exercise habits. Continue both your recreational activities and social pass times. These both contribute to your physical and emotional well being.
Be certain to get a good amount of sleep, especially the night before the test, because when you're overtired you are not able to perform to the best of your best ability.
Keep the studying pace to a moderate level by taking breaks when they are needed, and varying the work whenever possible, to keep the mind fresh instead of getting bored.
When enough studying has been done that all the material that can be learned has been learned, and the test taker is prepared for the test, stop studying and do something relaxing such as listening to music, watching a movie, or taking a warm bubble bath.

There are also many other techniques to minimize the uneasiness or apprehension that is experienced along with test anxiety before, during, or even after the examination. In fact, there are a great deal of things that can be done to stop anxiety from interfering with lifestyle and performance. Again, remember that anxiety will not be eliminated entirely, and it shouldn't be. Otherwise that "up" feeling for exams would not exist, and most of us depend on that sensation to perform better than usual. However, this anxiety has to be at a level that is manageable.

Of course, as we have just discussed, being prepared for the exam is half the battle right away. Attending all classes, finding out what knowledge will be expected on the exam, and knowing the exam schedules are easy steps to lowering anxiety. Keeping up with work will remove the need to cram, and efficient study habits will eliminate wasted time. Studying should be done in an ideal location for concentration, so that it is simple to become interested in the material and give it complete attention. A method such as SQ3R (Survey, Question, Read, Recite, Review) is a wonderful key to follow to make sure that the study habits are as effective as possible, especially in the case of learning from a textbook. Flashcards are great techniques for memorization. Learning to take good notes will mean that notes will be full of useful information, so that less sifting will need to be done to seek out what is pertinent for studying. Reviewing notes after class and then again on occasion will keep the information fresh in the mind. From notes that have been taken summary sheets and outlines can be made for simpler reviewing.

A study group can also be a very motivational and helpful place to study, as there will be a sharing of ideas, all of the minds can work together, to make sure that everyone understands, and the studying will be made more interesting because it will be a social occasion.

Basically, though, as long as the test-taker remains organized and self confident, with efficient study habits, less time will need to be spent studying, and higher grades will be achieved.

To become self confident, there are many useful steps. The first of these is "self talk." It has been shown through extensive research, that self-talk for students who suffer from test anxiety, should be well monitored, in order to make sure that it contributes to self confidence as opposed to sinking the student. Frequently the self talk of test-anxious students is negative or self-defeating, thinking that everyone else is smarter and faster, that they always mess up, and that if they don't do well, they'll fail the entire course. It is important to decreasing anxiety that awareness is made of self talk. Try writing any negative self thoughts and then disputing them with a positive statement instead. Begin self-encouragement as though it was a friend speaking. Repeat positive statements to help reprogram the mind to believing in successes instead of failures.

Helpful Techniques

Other extremely helpful techniques include:

Self-visualization of doing well and reaching goals
While aiming for an "A" level of understanding, don't try to "overprotect" by setting your expectations lower. This will only convince the mind to stop studying in order to meet the lower expectations.
Don't make comparisons with the results or habits of other students. These are individual factors, and different things work for different people, causing different results.
Strive to become an expert in learning what works well, and what can be done in order to improve. Consider collecting this data in a journal.
Create rewards for after studying instead of doing things before studying that will only turn into avoidance behaviors.
Make a practice of relaxing - by using methods such as progressive relaxation, self-hypnosis, guided imagery, etc - in order to make relaxation an automatic sensation.
Work on creating a state of relaxed concentration so that concentrating will take on the focus of the mind, so that none will be wasted on worrying.
Take good care of the physical self by eating well and getting enough sleep.
Plan in time for exercise and stick to this plan.

Beyond these techniques, there are other methods to be used before, during and after the test that will help the test-taker perform well in addition to overcoming anxiety. Before the exam comes the academic preparation. This involves establishing a study schedule and beginning at least one week before the actual date of the test. By doing this, the anxiety of not having enough time to study for the test will be automatically eliminated. Moreover, this will make the studying a much more effective experience, ensuring that the learning will be an easier process. This relieves much undue pressure on the test-taker.

Summary sheets, note cards, and flash cards with the main concepts and examples of these main concepts should be prepared in advance of the actual studying time. A topic should never be eliminated from this process. By omitting a topic because it isn't expected to be on the test is only setting up the test-taker for anxiety should it actually appear on the exam. Utilize the course syllabus for laying out the topics that should be studied. Carefully go over the notes that were made in class, paying special attention to any of the issues that the professor took special care to emphasize while lecturing in class. In the textbooks, use the chapter review, or if possible, the chapter tests, to begin your review.

It may even be possible to ask the instructor what information will be covered on the exam, or what the format of the exam will be (for example, multiple choice, essay, free form, true-false). Additionally, see if it is possible to find out how many questions will be on the test. If a review sheet or sample test has been offered by the professor, make good use of it, above anything else, for the preparation for the test. Another great resource for getting to know the examination is reviewing tests from previous semesters. Use these tests to review, and aim to achieve a 100% score on each of the possible topics. With a few exceptions, the goal that you set for yourself is the highest one that you will reach.

Take all of the questions that were assigned as homework, and rework them to any other possible course material. The more problems reworked, the more skill and confidence will form as a result. When forming the solution to a problem, write out each of the steps. Don't simply do head work. By doing as many steps on paper as possible, much clarification and therefore confidence will be formed. Do this with as many homework problems as possible, before checking the answers. By checking the answer after each problem, a reinforcement will exist, that will not be on the exam. Study situations should be as exam-like as possible, to prime the test-taker's system for the experience. By waiting to check the answers at the end, a psychological advantage will be formed, to decrease the stress factor.

Another fantastic reason for not cramming is the avoidance of confusion in concepts, especially when it comes to mathematics. 8-10 hours of study will become one hundred percent more effective if it is spread out over a week or at least several days, instead of doing it all in one sitting. Recognize that the human brain requires time in order to assimilate new material, so frequent breaks and a span of study time over several days will be much more beneficial.

Additionally, don't study right up until the point of the exam. Studying should stop a minimum of one hour before the exam begins. This allows the brain to rest and put things in their proper order. This will also provide the time to become as relaxed as possible when going into the examination room. The test-taker will also have time to eat well and eat sensibly. Know that the brain needs food as much as the rest of the body. With enough food and enough sleep, as well as a relaxed attitude, the body and the mind are primed for success.

Avoid any anxious classmates who are talking about the exam. These students only spread anxiety, and are not worth sharing the anxious sentimentalities.

Before the test also involves creating a positive attitude, so mental preparation should also be a point of concentration. There are many keys to creating a positive attitude. Should fears become rushing in, make a visualization of taking the exam, doing well, and seeing an A written on the paper. Write out a list of affirmations that will bring a feeling of confidence, such as "I am doing well in my English class," "I studied well and know my material," "I enjoy this class." Even if the affirmations aren't believed at first, it sends a positive message to the subconscious which will result in an alteration of the overall belief system, which is the system that creates reality.

If a sensation of panic begins, work with the fear and imagine the very worst! Work through the entire scenario of not passing the test, failing the entire course, and dropping out of school, followed by not getting a job, and pushing a shopping cart through the dark alley where you'll live. This will place things into perspective! Then, practice deep breathing and create a visualization of the opposite situation - achieving an "A" on the exam, passing the entire course, receiving the degree at a graduation ceremony.

On the day of the test, there are many things to be done to ensure the best results, as well as the most calm outlook. The following stages are suggested in order to maximize test-taking potential:

Begin the examination day with a moderate breakfast, and avoid any coffee or beverages with caffeine if the test taker is prone to jitters. Even people who are used to managing caffeine can feel jittery or light-headed when it is taken on a test day.
Attempt to do something that is relaxing before the examination begins. As last minute cramming clouds the mastering of overall concepts, it is better to use this time to create a calming outlook.
Be certain to arrive at the test location well in advance, in order to provide time to select a location that is away from doors, windows and other distractions, as well as giving enough time to relax before the test begins.
Keep away from anxiety generating classmates who will upset the sensation of stability and relaxation that is being attempted before the exam.
Should the waiting period before the exam begins cause anxiety, create a self-distraction by reading a light magazine or something else that is relaxing and simple.

During the exam itself, read the entire exam from beginning to end, and find out how much time should be allotted to each individual problem. Once writing the exam, should more time be taken for a problem, it should be abandoned, in order to begin another problem. If there is time at the end, the unfinished problem can always be returned to and completed.

Read the instructions very carefully - twice - so that unpleasant surprises won't follow during or after the exam has ended.

When writing the exam, pretend that the situation is actually simply the completion of homework within a library, or at home. This will assist in forming a relaxed atmosphere, and will allow the brain extra focus for the complex thinking function.

Begin the exam with all of the questions with which the most confidence is felt. This will build the confidence level regarding the entire exam and will begin a quality momentum. This will also create encouragement for trying the problems where uncertainty resides.

Going with the "gut instinct" is always the way to go when solving a problem. Second guessing should be avoided at all costs. Have confidence in the ability to do well.

For essay questions, create an outline in advance that will keep the mind organized and make certain that all of the points are remembered. For multiple choice, read every answer, even if the correct one has been spotted - a better one may exist.

Continue at a pace that is reasonable and not rushed, in order to be able to work carefully. Provide enough time to go over the answers at the end, to check for small errors that can be corrected.

Should a feeling of panic begin, breathe deeply, and think of the feeling of the body releasing sand through its pores. Visualize a calm, peaceful place, and include all of the sights, sounds and sensations of this image. Continue the deep breathing, and take a few minutes to continue this with closed eyes. When all is well again, return to the test.

If a "blanking" occurs for a certain question, skip it and move on to the next question. There will be time to return to the other question later. Get everything done that can be done, first, to guarantee all the grades that can be compiled, and to build all of the confidence possible. Then return to the weaker questions to build the marks from there.

Remember, one's own reality can be created, so as long as the belief is there, success will follow. And remember: anxiety can happen later, right now, there's an exam to be written!

After the examination is complete, whether there is a feeling for a good grade or a bad grade, don't dwell on the exam, and be certain to follow through on the reward that was promised...and enjoy it! Don't dwell on any mistakes that have been made, as there is nothing that can be done at this point anyway.

Additionally, don't begin to study for the next test right away. Do something relaxing for a while, and let the mind relax and prepare itself to begin absorbing information again.

From the results of the exam - both the grade and the entire experience, be certain to learn from what has gone on. Perfect studying habits and work some more on confidence in order to make the next examination experience even better than the last one.

Learn to avoid places where openings occurred for laziness, procrastination and day dreaming.
Use the time between this exam and the next one to better learn to relax, even learning to relax on cue, so that any anxiety can be controlled during the next exam. Learn how to relax the body. Slouch in your chair if that helps. Tighten and then relax all of the different muscle groups, one group at a time, beginning with the feet and then working all the way up to the neck and face. This will ultimately relax the muscles more than they were to begin with. Learn how to breath deeply and comfortably, and focus on this breathing going in and out as a relaxing thought. With every exhale, repeat the word "relax."

As common as test anxiety is, it is very possible to overcome it. Make yourself one of the test-takers who overcome this frustrating hindrance.

Additional Bonus Material

Due to our efforts to try to keep this book to a manageable length, we've created a link that will give you access to all of your additional bonus material.

Please visit http://www.mometrix.com/bonus948/nurseaceincare to access the information.